SAVING ELLEN

SAVING ELLEN

A Memoir of Hope and Recovery

MAURA CASEY

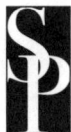

Skyhorse Publishing, Inc.

Skyhorse Publishing books may be purchased in bulk at special discounts for sales promotion, corporate gifts, fund-raising, or educational purposes. Special editions can also be created to specifications. For details, contact the Special Sales Department, Skyhorse Publishing, 307 West 36th Street, 11th Floor, New York, NY 10018 or info@skyhorsepublishing.com.

Skyhorse® and Skyhorse Publishing® are registered trademarks of Skyhorse Publishing, Inc.®, a Delaware corporation.

Visit our website at www.skyhorsepublishing.com.

Please follow our publisher Tony Lyons on Instagram @tonylyonsisuncertain

10 9 8 7 6 5 4 3 2 1

Library of Congress Cataloging-in-Publication Data is available on file.

Cover design by Kai Texel
Cover photograph by Getty Images

Print ISBN: 978-1-5107-8077-4
Ebook ISBN: 978-1-5107-8386-7

Printed in the United States of America

To the grandchildren of Jane Casey:
Anna, Tim, and Rachel;

And the great-grandchildren:
Ellie, Riley, Aiden, Angus, Arlen,
and all the generations to come.

Contents

Chapter 1: The Pickpocket   1

Chapter 2: Calling Cadence   5

Chapter 3: Play All Night, Work All Day   9

Chapter 4: The Projects: Fighting the Environment   13

Chapter 5: Moving to Anderson Place   21

Chapter 6: My Ellen   25

Chapter 7: The Island   29

Chapter 8: Kidney Failure   33

Chapter 9: The Professional Mourner   37

Chapter 10: The Paperweight   43

Chapter 11: The Affair   47

Chapter 12: The Limits of Prayer   55

Chapter 13: A Savior from Gary   59

Chapter 14: A Doctor's Curse   63

Chapter 15: Emergency Call from Gary   71

Chapter 16: The Inheritance   73

Chapter 17: Doddering on the Lake   77

Chapter 18: Booze, the Center of Life   83

Chapter 19: Starving for Survival   93

Chapter 20: Dialysis   99

Chapter 21: "Deadeye! Deadeye!"   105

Chapter 22: Bullies and Protests   111

CHAPTER 23: AFTER-SCHOOL CHOICES 119

CHAPTER 24: DALE'S LOT 123

CHAPTER 25: THE AFTERMATH 127

CHAPTER 26: THE SEARCH 131

CHAPTER 27: THE CURE-ALL ELIXIR 139

CHAPTER 28: WHEN TRANSPLANTS WERE MIRACLES 149

CHAPTER 29: PINING TO SAIL 157

CHAPTER 30: THE HOPE OF BUTTERFLIES 165

CHAPTER 31: THE TRANSPLANT 167

CHAPTER 32: STRETCH MARKS 171

CHAPTER 33: AREN'T GIRLS EQUAL? 181

CHAPTER 34: "WRITE. JUST WRITE." 187

CHAPTER 35: THE CAT AND THE PIT BULL 193

CHAPTER 36: RIPPING UP THE REPORT CARD 197

CHAPTER 37: THE MISSING PORK CHOPS 201

CHAPTER 38: THE BATTLE OF THE SKILLET 209

CHAPTER 39: PAYCHECKS AND POLITICS 217

CHAPTER 40: THE COST OF GIVING 223

CHAPTER 41: THE DIVORCE 227

CHAPTER 42: MONEY 231

CHAPTER 43: COACH, CHEERLEADER, OPTIMIST 237

CHAPTER 44: GASPING FOR AIR 245

CHAPTER 45: DELINQUENT 253

CHAPTER 46: ELLEN FINDS HER STRIDE 257

CHAPTER 47: MOTHER'S DAY 261

CHAPTER 48: SUMMER SKULLS 267

CHAPTER 49: A LAST SUMMER 271

CHAPTER 50: GOODBYES 283

CHAPTER 51: THE PRICE OF MOTHERHOOD 289

CHAPTER 52: PETE 297

CHAPTER 53: "IT'S DAD."   301

CHAPTER 54: ELLEN AND ELLIE   307

ACKNOWLEDGMENTS   313

TO MY READERS   317

BIBLIOGRAPHY   319

SAVING ELLEN

CHAPTER 1

THE PICKPOCKET

THE FLOORBOARDS GROANED. THE NOISE CRACKED IN THE SILENCE BETWEEN MY father's wheezing snores. I froze on all fours, in full view of Dad's mountainous form, my panic rising. Other kids might learn how to knit, or hunt, or cook, whether by family tradition or necessity; at eleven, I learned to steal from my father—and I was damn good at it.

With each step, the worn slats shifted, but the noise didn't wake him fully. He rolled over, restless, before his alcoholic gurgle resumed. My stomach tightened. Covered in blankets against the chill of a Buffalo winter, he was like a great hibernating bear and, for the moment, was sleeping like one. When I could breathe again, I crawled toward his sharp-creased suit pants hanging on the end of the bed. One pocket held bills folded into his money clip—the objects of my desire.

He had stumbled in the door as usual at 3 a.m. I heard him lumber up the seventeen stairs to my parents' bedroom. My mother sometimes slept elsewhere when he came in especially late, and that was the case on this particular night. She had her choice of rooms. There were plenty in the Victorian-era pile my parents had bought in 1964, four years earlier, for twenty-two dollars down and a handshake. The house on Anderson Place was our escape from the low-income housing projects where we'd languished despite Dad's management position at the American Red Cross.

A former rooming house, the home was in solid shape when we moved in. That didn't last. My mother used to say my university-educated father didn't know what end of a hammer to pick up. If something broke, he wouldn't know how to fix it and he was too cheap to pay anyone else. With six children living in the house, the structure soon showed signs of wear and tear. A hole gaped in the hallway wall from an errant elbow. Paint peeled outside. Plaster crumbled, and light fixtures drooped. Dad's drinking made him care less and less.

Worse, though, was how Mom worried about the bills. Money was scarce for even small things. Dad kept an iron grip on his paycheck and doled out money reluctantly. Mom had to plead with him for what little he gave her.

That's where I came in.

If Dad wouldn't give Mom the money she needed, I would simply steal it.

So, I crept around my parents' bedroom, measuring the pace of my father's heavy breathing. I reached the end of the antique sleigh bed and, ever so gently, lifted his pants from the footboard and lowered them to the floor. I felt around for the money clip and pulled it out.

$48—more than usual.

Here is where judgment came in. I had to take just enough to help Mom, but not so much that he would notice that the money was missing. Fourteen dollars seemed reasonable. I counted out the bills, then hesitated, barely breathing, feeling the weight of the coins in his pocket. Surely, he wouldn't miss some of those; what were the chances he counted his change before lurching to his car? It was worth the risk, I calculated. I counted out two dollars in coins, hung the pants up, and dropped in the money clip and coins.

Perhaps my hands were sweaty, or I wasn't as practiced at stealing loose change. But half the nickels, dimes, and pennies missed the pocket and scattered across the floor, breaking the silence between snores.

Dad woke up instantly.

"What the hell?" he growled.

Unable to see, he fumbled for his glasses, then reached for his pants. I slipped into the room I shared with Ellen. Her bed had been empty for more than a week. I dove under the covers and lay paralyzed, eyes clamped shut, heart hammering, as Dad came roaring down the hall.

"Who stole my money?"

He flung open the door to my room.

"Huh?" I said, pretending to wake up.

He ran down the hall looking in every bedroom, opening and shutting doors, awakening my bewildered siblings.

My mother was downstairs. She shouted up from the front hallway.

"Jesus, Casey, what on Earth is the matter?"

"Someone stole my money!" he bellowed. He stamped down the stairs to face my mother in the hallway. I crept out to watch the confrontation. Peering between the bannisters beside the stairs, I had a clear view of the front hall, eighteen feet below. She looked apprehensive, then she stiffened. She got angry, too.

3

"*We're* stealing your money? Fat chance. You must have spent more than you realized on your girlfriend last night," she said.

Each stared at the other, the silence between them hissed like a snake—long, menacing, and poisonous.

"I don't have to take this crap," he finally muttered, then he grabbed his coat and walked out, slamming the door so hard the whole house rattled.

I crept downstairs and stood beside my mother. We both watched my father through the window as he started his car, impatiently brushing off the newly fallen snow from the windshield. He flounced on the driver's seat and tore off. In silence, I handed my mother the bills and the coins. She took the money, still staring out the window. She said nothing, but her hands shook.

CHAPTER 2

CALLING CADENCE

"MOM, I'M COLD," I WHINED.

I was four and we were walking from the projects through the snow to the supermarket, a half mile away, while my brothers and sisters were in school. She bent down to me, smiling, took my hands to warm them in her own and began to sing, *Che Gelida Manina* ("What a Frozen Little Hand") from *La Boheme*, her beautiful operatic voice soothing me. Her knowledge of classical music and opera belied her family's working-class background; Mom had the Army to thank.

When everyone was home and the apartment fairly bulged with the activity of six children, Mom would call cadence when she needed a moment's peace. As the two youngest, Ellen and I were the most enthusiastic, becoming soldiers in an instant, marching around the living room and trailing one another around furniture as Mom rhythmically chanted out the beat of our footsteps while turning the pages of whatever book she was reading. Counting off as we marched was still effortless for her, twenty years after serving in the Army during World War II. She was a corporal but filled in for drill sergeants at one of the four bases where she served.

The Army introduced Mom to people and places far more diverse than her close-knit, blue-collar neighborhood in South Buffalo, an Irish enclave with a bar or a Catholic Church on every corner. Double-decker houses bookended the grain and steel mills that gave the region both pollution and prosperity. The smell of gas plants and burning ore lingered in the air. Women avoided putting the laundry out to dry when the prevailing wind sent soot their way. Yet, residents welcomed the war-fueled prosperity that finally reversed the economic downturn of the Thirties. Still, the scars from the Depression remained. My mother's family had lost their home to foreclosure. The tough times that followed, with its uneven meals, may have caused her lifelong heart murmur.

That whisper of heart disease was her father's justification for bursting into the Army recruiting office and blustering his objections after Mom enlisted in the Women's Army Corps. He had always been bitter that he had sired four daughters and no sons. But he saw his third daughter's decision to join the military as an act of defiance. It also meant that he would no longer get a portion of her paycheck from her job at Buffalo's Curtiss-Wright plant. The sergeant on duty retorted that Mom was old enough to make her own decisions, and that she would leave in three days.

Mom's decision was motivated by more than patriotism and rebellion. Only months before, she had survived a bout of encephalitis that left her delirious with fever for weeks. When she recovered, she wanted her life to mean something.

The Army became her great adventure. The two years she spent seeing the country shaped her, and in turn, her children. She became pals with members of the Army Band at Fort Oglethorpe in Georgia, who introduced her to classical music. Once out of the Army she used the GI bill to become the first member of her family to attend college, enrolling in the Great Books program at the University of Buffalo. She studied Greek, Latin, and French to read the classics in their original languages.

She took a sculpture course on a whim. While she waited for the teacher to arrive in class the first day, my mother took a lump of clay and in a few minutes created the figure of a woman weeping, her head in her hands. It reflected Mom's own grief. At the time, she had just lost her own mother and was deep in mourning. When the teacher saw her speedy work, she said she would cast the beautiful figure in lead and place it on a wooden pedestal so Mom could have it always. (It is now on my desk as I write.)

Sculpture, books, and classical music became my mother's passions. One more passion walked into Cole's Restaurant on Elmwood Avenue as she had a drink with friends. A black-haired stranger wearing a double-breasted suit, and a broad grin introduced himself. He said they had attended South Park High School together. Unimpressed, Mom said she didn't remember him at all. That fact would irritate my father for the rest of his life.

Chapter 3

Play All Night, Work All Day

DAD'S TEETOTALLING GRANDMOTHER WHO LIVED WITH HIS FAMILY KEPT A PITCHER of water ready by her bed, just in case she needed it.

She listened as Dad, then twenty, staggered up the stairs well after midnight after carousing with friends. She thought it was time drinking had more unpleasant consequences beyond a mere hangover. She gave him the gift of a few hours sleep, then walked into his bedroom and poured the icy bath from the pitcher over his inert form.

"If you can play all night, you can work all day. Get up!"

As he stumbled, gasping, out of bed, she handed him a list of chores. Nana helped shape his work ethic, but never successfully curbed his drinking.

My father grew up in South Buffalo, just two miles from my mother's childhood home, but in a world apart. He lived on a side street off wide, tree-lined McKinley Parkway, one of several sites an ever-penitent Buffalo named for the twenty-fifth president, who was assassinated in the city in 1901.

The Great Depression had no lingering financial impact on his family. His mother Bess was a public-school teacher. Dad's father, Bill, was a successful steel salesman. The commissions were generous, but the job kept him on the road.

So my father grew up surrounded by women. They alternately nagged and praised him, and cared for him through bouts of childhood asthma. Despite the ailment, he became a champion rower.

While attending the University of Notre Dame in 1943, my father joined the Army, smuggling in what he thought was enough asthma medicine to get through boot camp. He miscalculated. A day before graduation he had a massive asthma attack which sent him to Walter Reed Hospital for two weeks. The Army issued a medical discharge.

Gasping for air may have saved his life. Many of the GIs he had been destined to join died on the beaches of Anzio during the Allied invasion of Italy. Dad, meanwhile, weak and wheezing, caught a train to Arizona with instructions from his parents to stay long enough to regain his health.

The shift from the damp and cold Northeast to the clear desert air revived him like Lazarus. By the time the train crossed into Arizona, he was running up and down the aisles of the train, giddy and shouting, "I can breathe! I can breathe!" When the train rolled into Tucson, Dad hadn't felt so good in years. Even better: He arrived on St. Patrick's Day.

He grabbed his suitcase and walked across the street to the nearest tavern, which was mobbed. As Dad squeezed by revelers and inched toward the bar, he heard a female voice shout above the din, "Casey, you moldy son of a bitch!" It was a lively young woman he knew from college. A Tucson native, she had attended the women's college of St. Mary's, across the street from Notre Dame. She mischievously entered their names in a dancing contest that very evening. They won, and he stayed in Tucson for two years.

He might have stayed longer, but while visiting family in Buffalo, Dad's father laid down for a mid-afternoon nap on a snowy January day in 1945 and never woke up. His father's death set him adrift at the age of twenty-four, and he lingered in Buffalo. Then one day he walked into Cole's on Elmwood Avenue and saw Jane Murray, whom he remembered from South Park High School. He remained indecisive about a career, but he knew he wanted to be with Jane.

My mother always insisted that she married my father not merely for love, but because he was so persistent. He never gave up pursuing her, even when she dated others, even when his friends and fellow oarsmen in an eight-man shell wanted Dad to join their crew to help them qualify for the 1948 London Olympics. My father always said that he refused because he was afraid Mom would marry someone else while he trained. The crew lost the qualifying race by inches, he claimed. (Later, I found out that the closest any Buffalo crew came to qualifying was not losing by a whisker, but to place third.) In any case, Dad won his own contest. By the end of that year, he and Jane were engaged. He gave her a ring with a 1.5 carat diamond, the last remnant of his family's nineteenth-century wealth, one of two earbobs once worn by his great-grandmother.

The wedding was modest. The future seemed bright. Dad had a college degree, unusual for the time. The economy was booming. Buffalo in 1950 had 580,000 people. It was one of the most populous cities in the country, bigger than Dallas, with more than five times the population of Phoenix, whose growth was still in the future. The "Queen City of the Lakes" reveled in its importance as a critical shipping hub for goods on the way to the Midwest, as it had for decades. The opening of the St. Lawrence Seaway and its alternate shipping route from the Atlantic Ocean would add a one-two punch to the local economy. But that was still years in the future. At the century's midpoint, the area's thriving manufacturing base provided more than half of all city jobs. Factories such as Republic Steel, Pillsbury, General Mills, and the Trico plant struggled to keep up with the pent-up consumer demand after the Great Depression and rationing during World War II.

Despite the postwar prosperity, Dad drifted from job to job. The loss of his father had shaken his confidence. He sold insurance, and at one point sold cemetery plots on commission. The pressing need to support a wife, two boys, and four girls (babies that arrived almost every year) undermined the detached approach a good salesman cultivates.

"You can't make sales when you need the money," Dad said years later. "You lose all sense of timing. You push too soon. Customers can smell desperation. And they almost always walk away."

CHAPTER 4

THE PROJECTS:

FIGHTING THE ENVIRONMENT

THE PROJECTS, A CLUSTER OF SEVEN-STORY, DARK BRICK BUILDINGS, LOOMED over an area with no other apartment buildings. The edifices didn't have a neon sign blinking LOW-INCOME HOUSING, but they may as well have. We lived there for more than five years.

Surrounded by empty fields, the buildings and vacant expanse came with a cost. The price was the shattered hopes of Black and Brown people segregated by redlining, financial discrimination, and tradition on the East Side. City planners defended razing minority neighborhoods as the price of progress, calling it "urban renewal." They justified destroying the beautiful, two-hundred-foot-wide Humboldt Parkway, lined with elms and sycamores, for a six-lane highway that became Route 33 to help speed traffic from the airport and fuel suburban growth.

The projects overlooked the highway. The move wiped out part of Frederick Law Olmstead's plan for the city and devastated the lives of people with little power to object. When they protested, the city ignored them. The fields we played upon were made of bulldozed dreams. Each summer, the ice cream truck rolled through the neighborhood, with its tinkling jingle over and over, serving children on a street lined with projects, but devoid of homes or small shops that once stood there.

In the late fifties, the projects were not the graffiti-covered, trash-strewn slums they later became. But they were bad enough. Mom loathed the constant smell of onions and other fried foods from neighbors' apartments in the afternoon. She also hated the sound of neighbors' arguments in nearby apartments, the requirement that she mop the long hallway outside our living quarters as part of the rent, and the lack of access to a garden.

My father never told his co-workers where he lived. When my mother let that information slip at his office Christmas party, he was furious with her. She hadn't realized that he was keeping it a secret, but Mom, too, hated the fact that they lived in apartments for poor people.

While Mom was a night owl, rarely going to bed before midnight, Dad never needed more than five hours of sleep and was a classic lark, awakening early and cheerfully. To wake us up, he would jog down the hallway yelling, "Up tails! Up tails, all!" cribbing a line of poetry from Kenneth Grahame's *The Wind in the Willows*.

He would announce breakfast in stentorian tones, proclaiming, "Mother's Oats, made by father! Come and get it!" Mom gave baths, scrubbed floors, washed mountains of laundry, and cleaned. Dad rarely helped with housework. But it wasn't unusual for him to pitch in with an occasional meal and he always helped cook big holiday dinners.

My father, the morning optimist, was a storyteller; my mother, who must have been exhausted having had so many children in so short a period of time, had a rapier wit. She had a temper, but she rarely showed it and almost never lost control.

Mom had a long fuse, but when she finally gave into rage, legends were born. One grew out of an incident when my parents had only three kids. Dad found himself unemployed—again—and Mom reluctantly turned to her father, who allowed the family to move into his house to save money.

But Tom Murray was no genial patriarch. When he wasn't working on his prized rose garden in the backyard, he was drinking. When he wasn't drinking, he went out of his way to consume food and milk intended for the children. He delighted in needling my brothers, turning them against one another and inciting fights, which he then sat back and watched with a satisfied smile. My mom asked him to stop, but he sneered and refused, which sent her into an all-consuming rage.

Her thoughts turned to murder.

She researched methods at the nearby library and thought poison would do the trick. The best way, she decided, was to harness her father's innate gluttony and make the whole thing look like an accident. If she spoiled crab cakes, then chilled them enough to cover the smell, the greedy old man would see them in the refrigerator and eat them all. Nature would then take its course. Mom daydreamed of her father's poison-induced cramps, vomiting, convulsions, and fever. He would call out to her for help. She would feign concern. She would promise to contact the doctor, disengage the telephone, and leave with the kids for a day in the park, returning to find his lifeless form.

When she calmly outlined her death-by-crab-cakes plan to my father, he became so frightened that he borrowed money and moved the family within days.

Mom's heart murmur got worse. Finally, after my birth in 1957, succeeding bouts of pneumonia destroyed part of one lung. Doctors removed most of it, leaving her with a two-foot-long, white scar that snaked from her right shoulder blade down her back, curving underneath her rib cage. The incision and the muscles it tore open took a year for pain to subside. The angry, red scar eventually faded to white against Mom's freckled Irish skin. It made her so self-conscious she never wore a bathing suit again.

Exhausted after two miscarriages and six children, Mom brought up the subject of birth control. My devout father, knowing the Catholic Church forbade contraception, was dubious.

"We'll go to hell," he said.

"I'm in hell now," Mom replied.

Yet, birth control was not easy to obtain. The government had approved the Pill in 1957, but only to regulate menstruation. Every state had different laws. Some forbade the sale of birth control even to married couples. All the doctors known to Mom in Buffalo were Catholic. She thought it unlikely that they would help. She took a bus seventy-five miles to Rochester, where a friend arranged for her to obtain contraception from a Jewish doctor.

The babies stopped coming, but money remained tight. From time to time, Dad pawned Mom's engagement ring for ready cash. He always managed to buy it back before the pawn shop sold it to someone else.

After a string of jobs, Dad finally found a career he truly loved: working for the Buffalo Chapter of the American Red Cross. His storytelling, charisma, and outgoing personality enabled him to recruit throngs of volunteers to the organization. His career flourished, but we stayed in the projects, where my three sisters and I shared a bedroom and a mattress on the floor, and my two brothers shared a mattress in another room. My parents slept on a real bed in a third bedroom.

Mom played classical music to fight the environment. She would sing the soaring aria, "One Fine Day," from Puccini's *Madama Butterfly*, enchanting us with the story of Butterfly's broken heart. Mom scoured used book sales for children's editions on astronomy, Greek and Roman mythology, poetry, and fairy tales.

Her efforts paid off. Other than Ellen, who was bored by reading and always preferred running, jumping, or any activity over turning the pages of a book, the rest of us read constantly. On his first day of kindergarten, Tim told his teacher she was "obnoxious." She laughed later, telling our mother about Tim's use of a startlingly big word, the reason for his ire beside the point. I read the entire first-grade reader the first week of school. My wise teacher slowed me down by giving me a fourth-grade reader.

I lived in a bewildering forest of knees and legs. I was small for my age, and like most other cookie-cutter Caseys, had an Irish turned-up nose, dark eyes, and black hair like our father. Five out of six of us resembled Dad, a ratio that infuriated my mother. She needed no prompting at all to point out that she did all the work of bearing us and never failed to mention that labor, during all six bouts, was the most hideous, horrifying, excruciatingly painful experience of her life, perhaps close to crucifixion but certainly equal to medieval torture.

Our apartment felt like a small train station packed with hundreds of people coming and going all day long. My two brothers, Seamus and Tim, and three sisters, Claudia, Kate, and Ellen, began to refer to me as "the caboose." When we finally all sat down for dinner around the rough-hewn picnic table that served as our dining room table, I saw that we were only eight. It always surprised me.

As befit my placement in the pecking order, I felt loved, yet powerless. Seamus, as the oldest, took on parental responsibilities when they were out. When babysitting, he made up games that amused him and petrified the rest of us, like turning off all the lights to play haunted house and lunging at us from darkened corridors. He and Tim, who was less than a year younger, taught us to do the Twist, which Ellen and I did until we were dizzy.

Claudia, as the oldest girl, held sway over the younger three. She gave us written tests on manners before we visited relatives' houses to remind us to say "please" and "thank you," put napkins on our laps at dinner, and not to interrupt. I struggled over the questions, frowning in concentration. Claudia usually gave me an A for effort no matter how many questions I got wrong. Ellen would end up with a C, tear up the test, and run out to play. I ran behind her, ever the follower.

Seamus and Tim also taught us to fight, gifting Ellen and me tiny boxing gloves for Christmas when I was five and Ellen seven. I was terrified of violence. Ellen relished in the lessons. She hurtled herself into any conflict within or outside the family and usually threw the first punch. Mom refused to intervene, and responded to shrieks and loud accusations by yelling, "Don't call me unless there is blood!" When Ellen was eight, a boy shoved her at a nearby sledding hill, causing her to slip and break her wrist. The day after her arm was put in a cast, she sought out her aggressor and used the cast like a baseball bat, pounding him repeatedly.

Our brothers helped us navigate both school and neighborhood thugs like the Appenheimer Gang, so-called after a nearby avenue on which its members lived. But one gang in particular struck terror into the hearts of all the projects children. Its tactics were psychological rather than physical. Known as The Strippers, members threatened to rip off the clothes from any unwary child who walked in their neighborhood without permission, leaving the intruder to skulk home naked. Whether this was an empty threat or cold reality, the legend was effective. We avoided that area without fail.

Other gang members used brute force. My brothers began to get in fights regularly, including one memorable afternoon when several young toughs surrounded Seamus on his way home from school. During the fight that ensued, one slammed Seamus's head on the sidewalk. He was lucky to get out of the conflict with a concussion instead of a fractured skull. The threat and reality of violence signaled the end of our life in the projects.

CHAPTER 5

MOVING TO ANDERSON PLACE

MOM WROTE LETTERS REGULARLY TO HER AUNT LILLIAN AND WROTE TO HER with a request: "Please pray for us."

Lillian may well have prayed. But she was a practical woman, and she did more than plead with the Almighty. Within a week, Mom got a certified letter in the mail from Lillian's address in Gary, Indiana.

"Buy a house," the letter said.

Inside was a check for $3,000 for a down payment.

Mom and Dad settled on 145 Anderson Place on the west side of Buffalo, three blocks from Children's Hospital and two blocks from a library. The library sealed the deal for my mother. Yet the closeness of our house to the hospital would soon become vital for Ellen.

The house was just off the corner of Elmwood Avenue, a busy thoroughfare dotted with small shops and restaurants. The traffic became the soundtrack to our lives—a constant cacophony of sirens, screeching brakes, and honking horns. A cathedral arch of towering elms on either side of the street shaded the neighborhood. The trees were eighty feet tall, and each formed a leafy canopy two-thirds as wide. We took them for granted. Buffalo's grassy parkways and streets were lined with elms, so many that Buffalo was nicknamed the City of Trees. They made the most ordinary neighborhood beautiful, their branches so close together they nearly intertwined, forming a protective roof that cooled us in summer. In winter, the tree branches became the sheltering beams of a snow castle. Within a few years Dutch Elm Disease would kill them all. Beetles the size of grains of rice destroyed ninety thousand of the city's graceful, giant sentinels. Their destruction left neighborhoods like ours barren.

Ours would become the smallest of three large Irish families on Anderson Place. Two Palestinian families lived a few doors away. An Italian family lived across from the Palestinians. A childless couple from the then-Russian province of Georgia lived next door, crushing my hopes that a girl my age would be our nearest neighbor. The neighborhood stayed white until a Black couple moved in several years later, the closest our block came to being integrated.

The streets were our playgrounds. Our neighborhood had little green space aside from a bushy, tree-filled tract at the end of our street called Dale's Lot, which all the mothers in the neighborhood cautioned us to avoid. The nearest recreational space was two miles away. The kids played on the street, organizing kickball or baseball games, running to bases set up against the curbs. Others would stand in the middle of the street and send spiraling football passes high into the air. One kid would shout, "car!" and we momentarily scattered, seamlessly resuming play once the vehicle had passed.

One side of our house was adjacent to a service alley for a commercial building that housed a restaurant and a market. Traffic was constant from delivery trucks. When they left, rodents arrived, drawn by open barrels of grease from the restaurant and dumpsters overflowing with rotting vegetables just a few feet from our house. We adopted cats to keep the rat population down to manageable levels. The constant onslaught of cars was a death sentence for all but the nimblest feline. Few lived longer than three years.

Although the block crawled with children, I was tongue-tied when it came to making friends. That mattered less because Ellen was my daily playmate. Little did I know that her constant presence and companionship would soon end.

CHAPTER 6

MY ELLEN

"THIS IS MY DAUGHTER, ELLIE. SOMEDAY, SHE WILL BECOME THE FIRST WOMAN president of the United States."

My mother always said this with a smile when she introduced her fifth child to adults. She was only partly joking. It might have been the 1960s, but Mom knew that her daughter was going places. She was named Elizabeth Ellen, after Mom's grandmother. But everyone called her Ellie.

I alone addressed her differently. Early on, before the dawn of my own memories, I decided she might be Ellie to the whole wide world, but she was, and would always be, Ellen to me.

Ellen made friends effortlessly, especially with boys. She had no use for frills or dolls. When some misguided relative gave her a doll as a gift, Ellen would later pretend to be a pirate and make the dolls walk the plank or, worse, she would make a noose out of a rope and hang them.

Ellen loved male energy. Guys loved her because she was fearless, competitive, and eager to do what the boys were doing. When she wasn't playing with me, she shadowed our brothers, especially Seamus. At nine, she could throw a football nearly as far he could at fifteen.

Ellen preferred activity to reading. She was always on the move, and would challenge people to games constantly. Once, after practicing assiduously, she organized spitting contests. Ellen was a champion spitter, who taught me the dark arts of flinging saliva out of my mouth in an arc as far as eight feet, a socially inappropriate talent that I can still summon on command.

Ellen was as quick to cry as to laugh. I loved her, but I also feared her. She had Mom's temper without the long fuse, and packed a hell of a right hook.

Our squabbles often ended up with Ellen swinging at me. When she connected, as she usually did, my reaction was to hit the deck and shriek for Mom, who would tell Ellen to leave me alone. Most of the time Mom shrugged at fights, figuring that scuffles and the occasional split lip were inevitable. For my part, refusing to fight back was both a strategy and a reflection of my utter cowardice. Ellen was bigger and stronger, so whimpering and curling in a fetal position on the floor seemed a reasonable option. Fighting back never gained me the upper hand except for one occasion, where blind rage overcame my customary timidity.

This occurred when I was eight and Ellen was ten. We got into a shouting match at the top of the third-floor stairs. Ellen pulled back her fist and I reacted by shoving her, hard. She tumbled backwards down the stairs. Unsatisfied, I threw a chair after her. I landed in solitary confinement in our bedroom. My mother ordered me to tell my sister that I loved her and apologize. I didn't have an ounce of regret and figured the score was 999–1, in favor of Ellen. But I reluctantly complied—the price of getting dinner. Whispered threats from Ellen would make their way to my ears throughout the meal.

But I never doubted that she loved me. When I was in second grade and Ellen in fourth, a big sixth-grade boy began to chase me home for some real or perceived offense. Terrified, I sped past Ellen, who was walking with her friends, a half-block ahead. She turned around, sized up the situation immediately, and timed her next move. As the boy chasing me came near, she slammed her shoulder into him like an offensive lineman and sent him sprawling.

"Leave my sister alone!" she shouted. As the culprit scrambled up, he saw, not just Ellen, but her friends, mostly boys, standing behind her with arms folded, and hurried away.

In years to come I would miss that instinctive protectiveness. It was based, not just in her affection and loyalty, but in her enormous self-confidence and athleticism. The day would soon come when her self-confidence would wither along with her health.

CHAPTER 7

THE ISLAND

MOM DREAMED OF A PLACE TO GET AWAY FOR A FEW WEEKS THAT HAD ROOM for the kids to roam and places to swim. Buffalo, nestled in northern latitudes between Lake Erie and Lake Ontario, was burdened with gray skies and snowy winters during coldest months. But summer transformed Buffalo into one of the sunniest and driest cities in the Northeast, with more than fifteen hours of daylight. Affordable summer rentals abounded, particularly in nearby Canada.

Dad promised he would look for a summer rental. His "research" took him not to Lake Erie and Canada, but north to Lake Ontario. One night, he got drunk with an acquaintance, Tom Marin, who, in an alcohol-fueled bout of exuberance, told Dad to bring all of us to his summer cottage on East Cliff Island off Newcott, New York.

The next day, my parents drove the forty miles to Newcott. Tom, beer in hand, picked us up in a boat he had won in a poker game—an old, wooden runabout, painted bright yellow, appropriately named

The Banana Boat. Smugglers had once used the vessel to transport alcohol across the Great Lakes from Canada during Prohibition. We all fit on board for the short trip to the half-mile-long island. It had no streets for cars, just a crumbling sidewalk that bisected the middle of the island. At one end was a three-acre park, where the Marin cottage stood.

Tom's wife Peggy went ashen when we all trooped up the stairs from the dock and streamed toward the tiny blue cottage overlooking Lake Ontario. Tom hadn't bothered telling her that he'd invited an army for the weekend. They had five kids. Our family numbered eight. The cottage had three bedrooms, one bathroom, and a refrigerator which held a bottle of ketchup, three hot dogs, and a case of beer. My parents promptly went back into town, bought groceries, and returned.

We kids swarmed the property, swimming, playing in the grassy swale at the front of the cottage while the sun set over the water behind the small home. Ontario was deserving of its Iroquois language name, which means "Lake of Shining Waters." Nothing interrupted this vast inland sea. At night we gazed, awestruck, at the cloudy river of the Milky Way. The only sounds were the waves, the croaking of bullfrogs, and the wind in the trees. The experience was a stark contrast from our city home, with its wheezing buses, honking cars, and the incessant slamming and banging of delivery trucks. The air had no hint of engine exhaust or the cloying aroma of rotting produce from the dumpsters in the alley. Instead, the smell of fresh water mingled with the cut grass of neatly mown cottage lawns. At night, the lapping of the lake, the giggling of my sisters, and the sound of adults talking, laughing, and drinking on the porch lulled me to sleep.

THE ISLAND

In a first-ever extravagance, my father found the money to arrange a month-long rental of a cottage farther down the island from the Marins on the harbor side.

Our rented cottage overlooked the harbor, not the restless waters of Lake Ontario. Instead of the pounding waves, we awoke every morning to the bell-like song of wire halyards clanging against sailboat masts in the breeze. We did not own a boat, but that wasn't a problem. The Newcott brothers, descendants of the original English immigrant who founded the town, kept an ungainly fleet of mud-brown, large wooden rowboats tied up to the dock of the harbor's Spinnaker Bar, which they also owned. Anyone could rent a rowboat for $1 a day, or $60 for the summer.

The boats leaked. The oars were heavy. A motor was a luxury and out of the question. But we soon became adept at rowing and accustomed to the callouses on our palms.

Whenever Dad (or anyone else) needed a ride, they would order a beer at the Spinnaker, pick up the bar's phone and call on the party line to request that one of us row to the mainland and give them a ride to the Island. We became expert at navigating the sometimes-choppy water of the harbor to row the half mile to the Spinnaker. Otherwise, we spent our days fishing, swimming, and reading—borrowing books by the dozen from the small but well-stocked library in town. The cottage had no TV or radio.

And it was on the island, one day, that Ellen got a sore throat. She could hardly talk, but she refused to tell Mom about it. Mom, she told me, would take her temperature and make her stay in bed, even though she didn't want to. She wanted to fish and skip stones across the lake. She wanted to throw a football with our brothers. The sore throat would go away sooner or later.

Ellen and I wondered later on whether that terrible sore throat was a strep infection whose bacteria bobbed in her blood until it reached her kidneys, starting a chain of events that would change all of our lives.

Chapter 8

Kidney Failure

That September, our tans faded. We put away the tee shirts and denim shorts that were our summer uniforms and donned the green plaid skirts that marked us as elementary pupils of Cathedral School. As church-going Catholics enrolled in the parish, my parents only paid $10 for each of us to attend.

Ellen rarely complained. But some weeks after school began, she told our mother that she didn't feel well. She woke up one day with puffy eyes and swollen ankles.

As her symptoms worsened, my mother took her first to our pediatrician, then to an increasing number of specialists at the children's hospital three blocks away. Early on, she and Ellen walked there. My mother had never learned how to drive, a common occurrence in a city like Buffalo with a large mass transit system.

When Ellen wasn't at the hospital being poked and prodded ("They made me take my underwear off! I was so embarrassed!" she whispered to me one night in a half-sob), she was home. In the beginning, she welcomed time off from school. In the afternoons, she wanted to play and roughhouse with our brothers, but every time she did, our usually unflappable mother would snap at her to settle down. Soon, though, Mom didn't have to tell her to slow down anymore.

The other source of anxiety was Ellen's breath. It had an odd, ammonia-like smell because of the uremia swirling in her body that her struggling kidneys could no longer expel. She was producing less and less urine, and what she managed to produce looked dark. Soon the family learned a new word—*nephritis*, short for *glomerulonephritis*. The frightening disease was often a death sentence.

Kidneys measure around four to five inches long, yet they are marvels of sorting, sifting, dispersal, and absorption. They rid the body of toxins and their layers of filtration both extract and distribute the perfect combination of salts, water, vitamins, and minerals, keeping what is necessary and expelling what the body doesn't need.

But in Ellen, that delicate balance was disrupted. As the healthy operation of her kidneys waned, so did her energy, her optimism, and her loud, insistent spirit.

Confusion quickly swirled into chaos.

My parents always worried about a litany of things. We knew these specters by heart. Ellen hadn't been hit by one of the buses or trucks that, every few minutes, rumbled down nearby Elmwood Avenue, the reason Mom forbade us from owning bicycles. Ellen hadn't been in a fire, Dad's greatest fear, and the reason why we practiced fire drills at home. She didn't risk drowning, the threat of which made my parents insist that none of us swim alone ever, until we were at least twelve.

Instead, Ellen had a disease with a tongue-twisting name that had attacked an organ nobody thought twice about.

As Ellen's illness developed, with its constant hospitalizations, I felt an increasing sense of dread, accompanied by a faint sense of embarrassment. At my young age, I wanted to be like everyone else. Yet Ellen's condition set our family apart. Her condition made us abnormal. No one I knew had a family member under the age of fifty who was acutely ill, who went in and out of hospitals seemingly on a moment's notice. This slow-moving crisis, that I couldn't even explain to myself, was destroying not only Ellen's health, but our family.

Tension in the house mounted. My mother spent all day at the hospital. At home, she was distracted. When Ellen came home from her latest stint at Children's Hospital, she always seemed worse. She smelled faintly of the antiseptic that hung over the hospital hallways like a fog. She became anemic and exhausted, wilting before our eyes. No longer was Ellen loud and laughing, running to catch a football, demanding that our brothers play with her. For Ellen, who always wanted to leave the hospital and just come home, the house she returned to was not a lighthearted or welcoming place. Instead, everyone was sad.

For Dad, the situation worsened the feeling that he was being overwhelmed by worries and the responsibility of supporting people, which now included a desperately ill child.

CHAPTER 9

THE PROFESSIONAL MOURNER

IN THE ERA OF THE GREAT WHITE MALE, DAD HAD A COLLEGE DEGREE, UNUSUAL for the time. It is hard to understand why he didn't prosper more. His father's unexpected demise when Dad was in his twenties fueled his indecisiveness, and unemployment. Alcohol may have sapped his ambition. As more children came, there were more demands on his paycheck.

Dad exercised total control of the family finances despite my mother's offers to handle the budgeting. He complained about the bills so often that one day Ellen asked our parents if we were poor. They avoided answering.

Once he got steady work in a human service career he loved, he had a dependable paycheck. But financial worries didn't fade. He never felt that he matched the careers of his fellow Notre Dame graduates. His fortieth birthday upset him terribly and became the occasion for yet another bender. Finally, my mother told him to get a grip. She asked why his birthday was bothering him so much.

"I always thought I would have made my first million dollars by now," Dad replied.

My mother laughed.

He didn't talk to her for several days after that.

He would open the mail and mutter, "I'll never get ahead!" as he unfolded invoices for gas heat, lights, house insurance, taxes, and the $57-a-month mortgage payment.

Dad began the habit of giving me my allowance and then, a day later, asking me for the fifty cents back, saying he had bills to pay.

It was a request, not an order. He wheedled. He implied he was the victim of circumstances. He worked so hard. Times were tough. Every cent was crucial, didn't I see?

My father's request confused me. Whenever he would start asking me for the money back the familiar knots of tension would form in my stomach. *Do other fathers do this?* I wondered. Wasn't it bizarre for an adult to give children an allowance and then ask for it to be returned?

Still, I always gave back the money, until one day, I told my father in a low, furious voice I would spend every day working to grow up and earn my own money and I would never, ever ask him for anything ever again. Not just money. Anything.

He was horrified.

"That's an awful thing to say to a father," he said quietly.

He took the money but asked me to refund my allowance less often.

My father's insistence that we were edging ever closer to the poor house added a daily source of fear, and became the undercurrent of every conversation, the shadow in every room. Currency was not coins or paper; it wasn't merely a tool of trade or an extension of commerce. Money loomed large—an ancient, powerful, and exacting god, both an object of longing and yet somehow unattainable—dispensing confidence to those who had it and rendering powerless those who didn't. The latter of which I knew included us. As I grew, I knew I had to go to work as soon as I could to earn money that nobody could take away.

There were few ways for a kid to bring in cash. Babysitting normally would have been an option, but the families in the neighborhood were too large for the need to hire anyone. On the few occasions that parents treated themselves to a restaurant fish fry of Lake Erie perch or pike, or a dinner of roast beef piled high on a salty kummelweck roll served with a frosty Genesee Cream Ale, they relied upon older siblings to keep younger ones in check.

I was far too young to obtain "working papers." However, one job became available through the accident of our location. We lived across the street from a funeral home.

The funeral home was among the quietest businesses in our neighborhood. On funeral days, cars were double-parked along the street, starting in mid-afternoon for wakes, or in the morning, when employees would organize cars for a somber procession to the Cathedral two blocks away. When no funeral was scheduled, the employees would soap up and hose down the ebony-colored hearses and boat-sized Cadillacs until the chrome gleamed around the fin tail lights.

First, the undertaker, a tall, gaunt man named Warren Arthur, hired me to dust the golden oak woodwork of the funeral home, empty wastebaskets, and vacuum the green wall-to-wall carpeting once a week. After funerals, I shined the biers that awaited the coffins in the viewing rooms. I emptied the ashtrays overflowing with Lucky Strike butts and the slender, filtered cigarette butts of Virginia Slims favored by women and invariably stained with red lipstick. The pay was good—fifty cents for an hour's work.

Occasionally, Warren asked me to spend the night in the funeral home, in one of several apartments on the floor above the viewing rooms. He was too cheap to pay for an answering service, so his tenants were obliged to answer the telephone at night in case a body had to be transported from a hospital. When the tenants needed a night off, I took over. I had become accustomed to the presence of dead bodies, even dusting around them before wakes.

Warren had bigger things in mind for me than dusting, though.

At age ten, I became a professional mourner.

He saw me as the solution to a problem. Meager, grim funerals were bad for business. So, I showed up and performed at a moment's notice, my greed overcoming my shyness, whenever a scant crowd at a funeral needed a little pumping up.

Jocularity was not the goal. Funerals were not meant for a rollicking good time. Yet, larger funerals, with stories and conversation, and the occasional sip of whiskey from a flask discreetly offered and just as quickly tucked away, were what Warren and the men who worked for him preferred. The larger gatherings were springboards to more business, as relatives of the departed spoke of what a good job the home did. At smaller wakes, the families would nickel-and-dime Warren over the bill. They were less likely to tip the ushers.

In short, the sparser the funeral, the worse it was for business.

So, when a thinly attended funeral began to form, Warren would wait for his moment, and then address the group.

"There's a little girl across the street who was so moved—so *very* moved—by your loss that she asked me for a special favor."

Here, Warren would pause for effect, clear his throat, and say, "She would like to come in and say just a few prayers for your (mother, father, grandfather, grandmother, [fill in the blank here])."

The atmosphere would visibly relax. Adults would invariably smile and nod at each other, saying things like, "Isn't that fine?" and "We wouldn't want to stand in the way of a little girl's prayer, would we?"

I would come in, wearing the only dress I owned, one with little heart patterns, tied in the back with a bow. My face would flush with the attention. However, greed would overcome my normal shyness. Eyes glued to the casket, I would walk through the parting crowd and kneel before the coffin amid the scent of day-old flowers, then quickly cross myself, saying an "Our Father" and perhaps throwing in a "Hail Mary" for good measure. The object of my invocations—typically a withered, powdered old woman—rested with a slight frown, as if she knew that the whole charade was as empty as the grave into which she would soon be lowered.

I would then turn, and say, "I am *so sorry* for your loss." And sometimes I would give a little sniffle.

The adults would smile and nod to one another. Women would reach out and hug me as I wended my way through the crowd. And later, a smiling Warren would give me fifty cents for five minutes of work.

My mother and father thought it was the funniest thing they had ever heard, and didn't mind the deceit involved. I certainly wasn't about to let a twinge of conscience interfere with commerce.

Yet, too few skimpy funerals called for my services. I couldn't save enough coins to stop feeling the helplessness that a lack of money caused.

CHAPTER 10

THE PAPERWEIGHT

MY FATHER ALWAYS REFUSED TO WEAR A WEDDING RING. THIS INFURIATED MY mother because in the first decade of their marriage, she always wore hers. One day during an argument in the car, she yanked off her wedding ring and threw it at him. He ducked, and the ring sailed out the window. The issue was settled: From then on, neither of them wore a wedding band.

Dad's refusal might have been part of his desire to get away from his responsibilities, if only for a little while, my mother said years later. Her suspicion was confirmed one afternoon not long after we had moved out of the projects. My mother wondered what was taking my father so long to come home after work. She speculated to my brother Seamus, then a teenager, that he was lingering at The Place, a corner bar two blocks away that had been a neighborhood landmark since 1941. Seamus suggested that the two of them go and see.

They walked the short distance and entered the tavern where Dad was telling a story to a rapt audience. My mother greeted him gaily. Seamus followed, unmistakably his son; he looked like my father's younger twin. My father was visibly annoyed at their intrusion. Several bar patrons blanched, saying, "You never said you were married! And, you've got . . . *kids*?"

My mother laughed about it for years.

Dad had a ready excuse to his bosses if he were late; he held meetings at night to recruit volunteers. Once they signed up, he held evening classes to teach volunteers what to do in the aftermath of disasters. He needed help to cover fires, floods, and extend offers of aid to people rendered homeless. His insistence that he was invariably "at a meeting" if he was late became a family joke.

His Irish charm made him popular. And no matter how late he came home, he always went to work in the morning. If he was especially late, his secretary would turn on his desk lamp and scatter papers underneath so that it looked like he had just stepped away.

No one threw cold water on his alcohol use like his grandmother once did. And every adult we knew drank heavily from time to time.

This was, after all, the "Greatest Generation" that had survived both the Great Depression and World War II. Those searing experiences left most feeling entitled to a dinner of meat and potatoes along with what my mother called a "good, dark drink" of rye whiskey, (Fleischmann's if you were short on cash, or Canadian Club if you got a Christmas bonus). Those who preferred a glass of wine before going on to the real thing, that real thing being spirits, drank Wild Irish Rose, the pride of Canandaigua, New York—so sweet it was like drinking grape jelly.

Drinking was as much a part of life as the fashionable flock velvet wallpaper that covered the walls of every living room. Drunkenness was taken for granted until things got out of hand. Which, in our house, they did.

Seamus, the oldest, confronted Dad most directly about his drinking. He would argue with him about how little money he gave Mom.

"Mind your own goddamn business," he'd retort.

Seamus was taller than my father, and muscular, too, which gave him an imposing presence that could occasionally subdue my father.

One sunny afternoon, when I was around 10 or 11, a package from the Holy of Holies itself, the University of Notre Dame, arrived at our house. Dad opened it with great excitement. It was an ornate marble paperweight, weighing about a pound, with a brass plate on top. On the brass plate, beside an etching of the Golden Dome, was an inscription to my father, in gratitude for his service to his alma mater.

Dad was delighted. My mother was incensed.

"How much money did you give to Notre Dame for the good fathers to send you this?" she said.

My father looked innocent, then outraged.

"I gave of my time," he lied.

"Casey, I am not an idiot! Nobody gets something like this for volunteering!" my mother said, her voice rising. "Ellen needs shoes. Maura needs clothes. The house is falling down. And you're giving money to Notre Dame?"

The two of them traded barbs. Mom was sarcastic; my father, defensive. At one point, when the conflict seemed to be subsiding, I was in the living room, and my brother Seamus was sitting on the living room couch next to Mom. Our father was in the front hall, which opened up to the living room. Half to himself and perhaps to put the conversation on a more peaceful footing, he said, "What are we having for dinner?"

"Go eat the paperweight," Mom said.

Dad erupted, grabbed the chunk of marble, and threw it at my mother. It sailed in a direct line toward her face. She didn't have time to duck. I watched, horrified, frozen, knowing that the paperweight was a deadly weapon that was about to split open my mother's face in an eruption of blood and teeth. At the last possible moment, Seamus slapped down the paperweight in mid-air, and it fell harmlessly to the floor.

Silence. Then Seamus roared, reared up, and ran toward my father. He picked him up, flung him over his shoulder, ran up the stairs two at a time to our parents' bedroom on the second floor, and threw him across the room so he landed on the bed. Seamus then slammed the bedroom door shut and came back downstairs.

My father was intimidated enough that he stayed there for a long time.

Sometimes I wondered if he needed a fight to give him an excuse to leave the house and not come back for hours.

Ellen was an outlier, in that she adored Dad, but she was often hospitalized. As she got sicker, she wasn't there to witness many of the drunken scenes that began to occur with more regularity. Nor was she aware of my father's affair.

Chapter 11

The Affair

One of the couples with whom my parents socialized was Brigid and Jim Deland, the parents of nine children. They lived just a few streets away, and their children attended the same Catholic elementary school that we did.

When Brigid volunteered at our elementary school cafeteria, doling out shepherd's pie or fish sticks, she would sneak a few brownies sprinkled with powdered sugar onto my tray. She knew full well by the color of my lunch ticket that I had not paid the extra dime needed for dessert.

"Just between us!" she would whisper to me, and wink, as I blushed, happy with the attention and the unexpected treat. When she and her husband came over for dinner, she would take a few minutes to talk with us as though we, too, were grown-ups.

Sometimes, she went further.

The adults drank and talked long after my bedtime of 9 p.m. I could always hear them as I slipped into my nightgown. When I was about to drift off, Brigid would appear, silhouetted in the light of the hallway.

"Are you asleep?" she would whisper conspiratorially. She seemed to float over to my bed, exhaling a cloud of alcohol, a scent at once familiar and repellent. She would tell me that I was a wonderful girl with a beautiful personality and that she loved me best of all. I even outshone her own children. She would talk this way for several minutes, then kiss me before going back downstairs to rejoin the adults, leaving me wide awake, my heart pounding, thrilled and totally confused.

Could everything she said be true? No grown-ups noticed me. I knew my parents loved me, but they avoided complimenting children to avoid cultivating overweening egos. On the few occasions that I asked my mother directly, "Mom, am I smart?"

She would deflect, or answer so broadly as to render the reply meaningless: "Well, I think we all do OK in that department."

Yet, here was Brigid, slurring praise in the dark. Ellen was never in our bedroom when Brigid came in. Ellen was a little less than two years older than me and an unerring judge of people. She had noticed how Brigid lingered to talk to her, and me, on social occasions. Her behavior made Ellen suspicious.

"Why is she acting so nice? What does she *want*?" Ellen said.

I defended her. "What is wrong with being nice?"

Ellen frowned and shook her head. "I don't trust her."

Ellen was right, but it took another year or so for the rest of us to see past the veneer of Brigid's kind words and the manipulation that slithered beneath the surface.

One weekend, my parents invited Brigid, who came without her husband, and another couple to East Cliff Island. Following an afternoon of drinking, Dad, Brigid, and the couple decided to swim. My mother, ever conscious of the long scar from her lung operation, avoided swimming, so she stayed at the cottage.

After that weekend, we never saw Brigid in our home again. All contact stopped. I felt deserted. Brigid liked me. She liked all of us. She was nice. Why couldn't we see her?

Years later, we found out that swimming was not all that took place that night on the beach. The other couple quickly left in disgust and told my mother. The affair soon became an open secret, gossip passing from one neighbor to another.

Us kids began to suspect something was up when Dad, a devout Catholic with an instinctive reverence for the clergy, began to complain about the pastor of our church, Father Garvey.

He wasn't any damn good. His sermons were mush. He asked for money from the pulpit too often. My father's complaints confused me. *Father Garvey was a nice man*, I thought, and always gave those of us at the Catholic elementary school a half day off on March 17, St. Patrick's Day. Who could object to kind Father Garvey?

Dad railed against the priest not because of his sermons, but because of what happened when he and Brigid attended Mass together. They approached the altar to receive communion, and Father Garvey noticed their hands touching as they knelt. He perceived the situation instantly and skipped over them, refusing them the sacrament.

Dad and Brigid thought the priest had made an error, and remained at the altar rail, which soon filled with other parishioners who knelt around them, awaiting the host. Father Garvey came back down the line of parishioners, placing the wafers on tongues, but once again skipped over Dad and Brigid, ensuring they both got the message. Being denied communion enraged my father.

The public nature of his affair resulted in some trying to shield my mother, my siblings, and me from embarrassment.

Every Christmas, our street's legendary social event of the year took place: the Bennetts' all-night Christmas Party. The party began early Christmas morning around 1 a.m., after Midnight Mass concluded at the cathedral, and continued until 5 a.m. The event featured a Bacchanalian feast, festive music, and drunken carol singing. Heaven help the parent who, beleaguered with alcohol and bloated from overeating, still had toys to assemble before dawn. My parents avoided this by allowing us to open toys on Christmas Eve, dissolving the myth of Santa Claus.

At one such party, neighbors surrounded my mother and me in the Bennetts' kitchen. Whenever we tried to move into the living room, someone would ask me about school or sit my mother down and put a drink in her hand. After a while, Mom would try to get up and John Bennett himself would insist she stay.

"Jane, you have such a lovely voice," he said. "Won't you lead us in Christmas carols?"

That continued for an hour and a half. Later, we found out the real reason for the constant interventions. My father was nuzzling Brigid in another room. Finally, someone asked him to leave the house, which he did. When the coast was clear, Mom and I could circulate once again.

Every family has its secrets. Like a string of firecrackers going off, one by one, each one of us found out about the affair in our own way. Claudia's revelation at fourteen was tinged with malice. A single woman in her forties lived across the street from us. Ann Steppen took it upon herself to nonchalantly tell Claudia that her dad was having an affair. Claudia said nothing. Afterward, she went home and vomited.

My discovery was accidental. I was in eighth grade and mentioned to my mother that Dad was coming home even later than usual.

"He must be having an affair," I joked.

"Oh, I didn't realize that you knew about Brigid," Mom replied.

I stared at her, and then moaned and doubled over as if someone had punched me. I saw everything in an instant—not merely my father's betrayal of my mother. At once, I realized that my father's penury was not because he didn't make enough money. He denied our needs to tend to his girlfriend's desires.

Their trysts included the oddest rituals. Brigid and my father did their families' grocery shopping together, competing over who could save the most at the local A&P. We all noticed the declining quality of our food. Sometimes the meat, drastically marked down, would have a slightly greenish tinge. Lettuce wilted. Milk, and the cost of it, was an ongoing issue since the happy couple had fifteen kids to feed between them. We mostly drank powdered milk mixed with water, and a little whole milk added to make it more palatable. But Dad never stopped complaining about the cost of dairy and, I suspect, neither did his girlfriend.

Dad and Brigid figured out that a vending machine that dispensed half gallons of milk had the cheapest prices. That big, dirty, white, vending machine in front of a row of stores became their rendezvous point, and an irresistible family joke. We made up songs featuring that most romantic of all settings—a beat-up fridge at the edge of a crumbling parking lot.

My siblings and I united in guerrilla warfare, particularly against my father. It wasn't because he drank too much or that he ignored the increasingly dilapidated condition of the house, with paint peeling and a porch so rotted that even the mailman complained. It was because he was spending as little as possible on the family to spend as much as he could on Brigid.

Like starlings forming a murmuration, we six kids acted individually and in tandem. Tim, the second oldest, tapped into his love of Greek and Roman mythology. He refused to call Brigid by her given name and dubbed her Circe, which the others found hilarious. I didn't get it. Finally, he patiently explained that Circe was the Greek nymph in the Odyssey who turned men into pigs.

Perfect. We rarely used her real name again.

Next, we took aim at our father's pride in being a graduate of Notre Dame. Western New York alumni of the school bestowed upon Dad its Man of the Year award in 1963 at an elaborate annual banquet where attendees basked in the glow of their shared collegiate experience. The ornate proclamation his brother alumni gave him was signed by the president of the university, topped by an etching of the Golden Dome, outlined in Virgin Mary blue, and surrounded by a wooden frame of painted gold. Ever after that special night, it hung in the front hallway of our home.

Naturally, it became a target of our growing hostility.

When Dad went on a bender, he would enter the house and find that his award had a drunken tilt. Cursing, he would straighten it. The next day, it was crooked once again. Straighten, tilt; straighten, tilt. The thing began to have a permanent list like the Tower of Pisa. Finally, it disappeared from the front hall altogether. One of my siblings hammered a nail in the drywall next to the toilet and there hung the award—at a rakish angle—for all to admire.

Dad yanked the award off the wall and put it in his bedroom.

Claudia got him back one day when, after a particularly heavy night of drinking, he got a powerful case of the runs. Our house had one small bathroom. There had been a working second bathroom in the basement, but as it fell into disrepair, my father never got it fixed. This came back to haunt him when he became overwhelmed with the call of nature and ran down the hall to the bathroom shared by all, only to find it occupied at that moment by my sister. He began to pound on the door. "I need to get in! Hurry up!"

Claudia replied, in a tone of exaggerated politeness, "Really? *Whatever* could be the matter?"

"I've got the runs! Open the goddamn door!"

"I am so sorry, father. I am indisposed at the moment."

"For Chrissake, hurry up! Hurry! Hurry!"

"I heard you, father, and I wish to assure you that I am moving just as quickly as I possibly can. It will just take a few more moments of my time."

Erupting in obscenities, Dad ran downstairs and out the door—to the gas station a block away, where, presumably, he found relief in its public bathroom.

What kept my father from becoming a monster, from eliciting only fear, was a truly unusual quality. He could not hold a grudge for more than sixty seconds. He would get angry. His behavior when he was drinking was frequently unforgivable. But he never stayed mad. When his anger blew over, it was done. Then he acted like nothing happened at all.

CHAPTER 12

THE LIMITS OF PRAYER

MY FATHER ESCAPED HIS DISAPPOINTMENT AND WORRY IN DRINK, WHILE MY mother sought solace in prayer, which sprang from her own deep faith.

She rarely attended Mass on Sunday morning, as it was one of the few hours in the week when she got some peace and quiet. When we were very young, our father took us all, and we followed him like ducklings down the center aisle of the invariably packed church. When we were older and had moved to Anderson Place, we walked the two blocks to St. Joseph's New Cathedral to attend the 9 a.m. children's Mass. It was no different from any other Mass, except ever-watchful nuns, who, like prison guards, took note of pupils who were present and those who were not. The slackers would face the Sisters' wrath come Monday morning.

Mom was even less likely to go to Mass when, in the late 1960s, the Vatican changed the liturgical language to English from the Latin she loved. The few times we attended Mass together in the immediate aftermath of Vatican II, she still refused to go along with English.

She was equally stubborn when evangelicals would come to our door intent on converting the non-believers in our home to their born-again version of Christianity. She handed them her Greek language edition of the New Testament, explained that the Gospel of St. Luke was originally written in Greek, to the horrified missionaries, and suggested a discussion on the accuracy of their bible's translation. The visitors would leave quickly.

She may not have gone to weekly Mass, but she prayed every morning for about twenty minutes, during which we knew better than to bother her. Each day she opened a well-thumbed prayer book and soon entered a meditative state, softly whispering as she read, momentarily oblivious to the household noise around her.

We had few crucifixes in the house, but on a white table on the landing of the back stairs stood a large, yet simple statue of baby Jesus that had once been an Infant of Prague, complete with its characteristic ornate robes. One day, a woman brought the original ceramic statue, in pieces, to my mother in her sculpture studio and told Mom it had been in her family for years and she could not bear to throw it out. She left the shattered statue with Mom, who took months to repair it, forming it into a far simpler version of the original. The woman never returned, so Mom brought home her version of a young Jesus—a crowned, sturdy boy in a simple white robe with a faint smile.

A little sign before the statue read, THE MORE YOU HONOR ME, THE MORE WILL I BLESS YOU.

The phrase always made me wonder how God could truly be omnipotent if He required praise as payment before answering prayers. The statue was usually illuminated with the flickering

light of a votive candle that my mother kept lit. It became her preferred symbol of Christianity—not the tortured Christ of the cross,
but a child, one far more serene and placid than we ever were.

Mom believed prayer could do anything. As a teenager, she seriously considered becoming a Carmelite nun, joining the walled-off
order of Sisters in the monastery of the Little Flower of Jesus in
North Buffalo. Taking final vows would mean a life in seclusion, of
sleeping on a straw mattress, wearing a heavy brown woolen habit
and rope sandals, and making the choice to rarely see her family.
Instead, she would live in community and pray for hours each day.

She was ready to dedicate her life to meditation, manual labor,
and silence, but her mother talked her out of joining. As time
passed and children came, she put her faith in those few moments
every day when she communed with the Almighty.

"Prayer moves mountains," she would say, and we knew she
believed it.

Mom saw God in every vein of every leaf, in sunrises, in kittens
and small acts of kindness. Her spirituality was so vivid, her faith
so strong, that there is no doubt she threw herself into prayer when
Ellen became ill.

She waited for an answer and a glimmer of hope.

CHAPTER 13

A SAVIOR FROM GARY

WE REALIZED THAT ELLEN'S SITUATION WAS SERIOUS WHEN AUNT LILLIAN, whom we'd only heard stories about, announced that she intended to visit.

My mother boarded a Greyhound bus to visit her once every several years, a welcome respite from all of us. In a few weeks, Mom would return, looking rested, with small presents packed in her suitcase.

Mom encouraged us to write letters to her beloved aunt, even though none of us had ever laid eyes on her. But we knew her importance to our family, and of her love for our mother. We wrote long letters on the backs of rolled-up strips of wallpaper, spare from when my mother redecorated several rooms. We rolled the long scrolls in tubes, which upon arrival made her laugh and gave her something to unfurl dramatically to her friends. They might brag about their grandchildren, but the childless Lillian had attentive nieces and nephews who wrote her letters six feet long. Top *that*, she implied.

The plan was for Aunt Lillian to help Mom handle the chores and give her more time to spend with Ellen, shuttling her from doctor to doctor and to Children's Hospital, where there were always more tests. We finally would meet the woman from the Midwest to whom we had written, the one who gave solace to our mother like nobody else, and yet who remained a mystery.

While we waited for her arrival, we were unnaturally quiet, all sitting together in the living room, most of us pretending to read.

Finally, the front door was flung open and Lillian stepped into the front hall, wearing clip-on blue earrings and a mink stole and saying, over and over, "How-DEE! How-DEE!" with a flat, midwestern twang. The room exploded in shouts as we surrounded her in welcome, taking her bags from Dad and helping her take off her mink. Within moments of setting foot in the house, she donned an apron. A broom rarely left her hand. When she wasn't cleaning, she was cooking.

Lillian's specialty was her lemon meringue pie. A bowl full of fresh lemons and bags of flour and sugar at the ready, she would seemingly spend hours rolling out dough and beating egg whites into fluffy clouds that were unrecognizable from their original form. Her pie was an unending source of wonder to my brothers and sisters; one spoonful made them feel glad to be alive. Lillian was delighted with the reception, so she made more.

Everyone was thrilled, but me.

I didn't like lemons. Too tangy. I tried the tiniest bit of pie, and didn't like it.

The reaction from the rest of the family was something on the order of, "What are you, a communist?" Soon, however, they realized that my meringue boycott left more for them. No pie? No problem.

Lillian was bemused, then amused. I was apparently the first person in history who could resist her signature dessert that inspired paroxysms of joy in everyone else. She didn't insist that I try "just one bite," like other adults, instead accepting my unwillingness to compromise. She may have had some of that same stubbornness herself.

Lillian rarely talked. Cooking and cleaning were how she showed affection. She exuded an abruptness I wasn't accustomed to in women. Cuddly, she was not.

One day, wielding her broom, her ever-present apron tied in a bow at her waist, she signaled with a crook of her finger that I should come closer. The apron's pockets hung loose from wear.

"Put your hand in there," she commanded, pointing at her left pocket. I was mystified. What could it be? *Nothing good*, I thought. *Maybe a spider?*

I was wary, equating her gesture with Seamus's pranks. He routinely hid candy bars in his desk drawer under mouse traps that snapped my tender fingers when I tried to sneak a piece of candy.

Apprehensive, I put my hand into her pocket, then yanked it out.

"Do it again," Lillian commanded. I put my hand in, then just as quickly, pulled it away. Lillian became exasperated.

"Put your hand in there and *pull out what you find*," she snapped. I closed my eyes, put my hand in the cavernous pocket, and pulled out a tube of rolled up dollar bills.

My eyes widened. It was more money than anyone had ever given me at one time: $3.

"It's your birthday next week," Lillian said gruffly. "Buy something." As I stood stunned, she turned away and continued sweeping.

Within a few weeks, Lillian was gone. She had cleaned the house from top to bottom, cooked some dinners ahead and put them in the freezer. Her presence was both practical and a source of comfort for our mother. We never saw Lillian again. But her influence would soon change all our lives, just as it had when her intervention rescued us from the projects.

CHAPTER 14

A DOCTOR'S CURSE

ELLEN HAD SOME DAYS WITH MORE ENERGY, WHEN I CAUGHT GLIMPSES OF THE lively sister who was fast fading from my memory. But generally, her health continued its slow decline. Often when a test came back with poor results, her doctors would admit her to the hospital three blocks away. Ellen was usually on the fifth floor, and I couldn't visit. The rules were strict: nobody younger than fourteen could enter patient floors. The few times I tried, nurses instantly intervened, as if I were trying to break into the Vatican. Their vigilance meant the only way I could see my sister was to walk three blocks to the hospital and, at the appointed time, wave at her room from the parking lot below. She would signal back, opening her window a crack and waving her hand frantically. It was frustrating and even a little ridiculous, but the only solace available to us.

During her stays, nurses told Ellen she could stay in pajamas all day if she wanted, but she refused. She wanted to feel normal, so she would get up in the morning and change into jeans and a shirt, like she would at home.

She would read books Mom brought her, if she felt well enough. Buffalo's public school district sent a tutor to help her keep up on schoolwork, and she worked on lessons when she could. In between tests, she played endless games on a wooden tic-tac-toe board.

Every day, Mom appeared at the hospital, gently teasing Ellen, brandishing a pack of cards and challenging her to a game of rummy. They always kept score. Ellen won frequently enough that Mom sometimes accused her of cheating, then they would laugh and play again.

Yet, other times Ellen wouldn't feel well enough to play. Her kidneys poorly regulated her blood pressure, and it soared. Headaches plagued her constantly and exhaustion sapped her vigor. Medications that helped everyone else never seemed to work as intended. Penicillin gave her hives. Other pills caused unpredictable side effects.

As time passed, Ellen grew increasingly upset, and card games couldn't distract her. She didn't feel well, but she was sick of being in the hospital. She missed her brothers and sisters, and our cats, and our Beagle mix, Sam.

She wanted to go home.

At first, Mom tried to kid Ellen out of her bad mood. But nothing she said helped. Finally, Mom sighed and put aside the cards, sat next to Ellen, and told her the truth: She was *really sick.* And she couldn't go home until the doctors gave their permission. She didn't know how soon Ellen would get better, or when the day would come that she would be healthy and feel normal again, when she could put behind her the bad memories of hospitals, needles, tests, and feeling terrible. While new treatments were invented every day, nobody could predict the future.

"So, you have a choice," Mom told Ellen. "You can whine through this illness and stay mad. And honestly, no one would blame you. We all know this is scary and hard. But, complaining won't make you feel better. Not for a minute."

Ellen listened intently, silent, in the spartan hospital room. The houses five stories below were a checkerboard of shingled roofs and tiny lawns, reflecting sun and the shadows of clouds.

"You also have another choice," she continued. "One that comes more naturally to you. You can be brave. That doesn't mean that you will feel less scared or mad that this happened. It does mean that you will try to make it through all this with as little complaining as you can manage. It won't make the symptoms go away, but it will make you feel better in the long run." She paused, putting the cards in her purse, and picked up her coat.

"It's your life. It's your choice, and I am just as sorry as I can be that this is how things are turning out."

Mom left the hospital and walked home.

Ellen thought about what our mother said and decided that she would try to meet every test, every awful symptom, without complaining. She would figure out a way to endure. Her way.

And so she did.

When things felt particularly grim in the hospital, Ellen would pretend to be a prisoner of war. She would set aside the silverware and eat her small meals with her hands.

She would play practical jokes. Our brothers and their friends brought her rubber toads and snakes, and she flung them at the nurses, who were profoundly unappreciative. But their startled reactions made Ellen laugh.

Thirst overtook her as doctors restricted her liquid intake to ease pressure on her ailing kidneys. Ellen turned her deprivation into a game. Between those glorious moments when Ellen could drink, she pictured she was on a deserted island, searching for a spring to survive another day until a rescue ship appeared, or trudging through the desert, a member of the French Foreign Legion, forced to ration what little water she had to drink. For who knew when the next oasis would appear on the horizon?

When her imagination failed to take her mind off her thirst and she could stand it no longer, Ellen would pour an ounce or two of the precious liquid. She'd roll it slowly around her mouth until at last it trickled down her parched throat. Soon cravings for more would start again.

Plotting her escape, Ellen began to keep track of nurses' shifts, especially the supervisors. Ellen knew deep down she really couldn't sneak out of the hospital. Even finding the strength to run the three blocks home seemed out of reach. But she dreamed of a jail break, mapping the precise number of steps it would take to get to the stairs, and calculating how long it would take to go down the five flights and slip away during shift changes when the staff was distracted.

Her reaction to her illness shaped her sense of humor.

When visitors or doctors asked "Ellen, how do you feel?" she would pause, and say, "With my fingers."

Ellen was the same way when she came home from the hospital. She pushed everything behind the curtain, never revealing how frightened she was or how long and dark the hospital nights seemed, far from the people and things she loved.

Mom was openly proud of Ellen's response to the illness, her refusal to complain, her sense of humor, and her growing determination to act as though nothing was wrong.

"That's my Ellie," Mom would say.

Other times, she would say, "You've got to leave them laughing. Stick it out. Don't, for God's sake, whine."

And yet, Ellen's courage—part denial, part determination, always shielded by a hardened shell of relentless humor—became the unspoken standard for the family. It became both our pride and our albatross. Our complaints felt trivial. I felt as though I couldn't talk about things that upset me. Ellen's refusal to complain, and my mother's pride in her example, by implication, denied the rest of us the right to complain or to admit that anything was wrong.

Mom didn't want anyone outside the family to know the details of what Ellen was going through. Neighbors, friends, and relatives already understood she was sick, an unavoidable consequence of how many weeks of school she missed and how often she was in the hospital. When people asked me how Ellen was, I learned the best response was, "She's doing as well as can be expected," a meaningless statement by any measure.

While it prevented gossip, it also cut off any opportunity for others to offer emotional support. Within the family, we almost never talked about how terrible we all felt, or how worried we were. The determination to act as though everything was OK, or would be, guaranteed that, most of the time, we couldn't support one another.

Once in a while, though, reality broke through.

On one cloudy afternoon, I walked home from fifth grade to find my mother home instead of visiting Ellen in the hospital. As I put down my books, I sensed something was wrong. She seemed strangely quiet, and didn't greet me. From the front hall, I could see her sitting in the living room, staring into space. Mechanically, her head turned toward me at the sound of my greeting. Her face was pale, drawn.

"Maura," her voice shook. "Dr. Hardy told me today that Ellen will die before she turns eighteen."

Mom had gone to see him because she wanted a clearer prognosis concerning Ellen's illness. She wanted her Ellie back—the girl who once exuded high spirits and now was quickly becoming a distant memory. She wondered when all the treatments would have a positive effect.

Dr. Hardy sighed, and told her that all the treatments were just delaying the inevitable.

Ellen's disease was always fatal. Already, specialists struggled to slow its progression. Dr. Hardy could not envision any plausible scenario in which Ellen would live to adulthood.

"Enjoy your daughter while you can," he said, shaking his head. "Be grateful you have a big family. You have other children. Take comfort in them."

This was 1967. Kidney transplants, now so ordinary, were then still so rare, almost experimental. Kidneys were the first human organ to be transplanted, starting in the mid-fifties, but the operation usually didn't work for long.

Renal disease treatment, at the time, amounted to trying everything to stall the illness in the hopes that new drugs and treatments would come along. Delay was the name of the game. It bought time, little more.

Dr. Hardy was blunt. Barring a miracle, my sister's days were numbered.

I was outraged at the doctor, panicked at his message, and determined to comfort my mother all at the same time. What did the doctor know, anyway? I argued. Could he see the future? And Ellen might beat the odds.

"Everything will be all right," I said. "You wait and see."

My mother looked at me in gratitude, then she crumpled in guilt. "I shouldn't have told you," she whispered. "Now you'll worry."

I told her it was OK. It wasn't, of course.

Now I knew how sick Ellen really was and how dim the hopes were for her recovery. She might never again throw a football with the boys.

Consumed with dark thoughts, I pushed them away.

I couldn't—wouldn't—believe that Ellen would die. *She would get better*, I thought. *She had to. Someday, everything would be made right again.*

Chapter 15

Emergency Call from Gary

One September afternoon, I watched my mother water the two backyard Kwanzan cherry trees she had planted, along with a few struggling shrubs near the chain-link fence that now gave us a sweeping view of the parking lot.

Our small, pretty courtyard was gone when the theater that walled it in was torn down, but Mom clung to her vision, nonetheless. Large stones were stacked in the hopes that someday Dad and the boys would lug them into place and she could piece together a Japanese rock garden. But nobody ever made the time.

Suddenly, the phone rang, disrupting my thoughts.

"This is an emergency call from Gary, Indiana, for Jane Casey." I shouted the message to my mother.

Mom dropped the hose, still spewing water, and ran into the house.

Lillian had died, unexpectedly, at the age of eighty, during a minor operation. Her heart stopped, and medical personnel could not revive her. Our mother's kind and steadfast comforter was gone.

Mom left for Gary. Dad stayed at home with us. We were left to contemplate what Aunt Lil meant to our family.

Maybe I should have given her lemon meringue pies more of a chance, I thought. She always scared me a little, yet she was the closest thing I had to a grandmother. Dad's mother had died when I was six, and Mom's had died before her marriage. My parents each had sisters with children, but they were all busy raising their own families and we almost never saw them. Now there was one fewer relative, and nobody to write to anymore.

Mom was in Gary for more than a week and said little about the funeral, except for a scene that struck her as so evocative, and so courteous.

As the funeral procession, led by the hearse, made its way to the cemetery down Gary's quiet streets, she noticed three men going to work, each carrying lunch boxes and loudly joking with each other. They were all laughing until they noticed the hearse and small line of cars following. The men stopped talking, and as one, they all removed their hats and stood with quiet respect as the slow line of cars passed.

My mother, the lead mourner of a tiny funeral to bury an elderly lady with almost no other relatives, was moved by the grace of strangers. She felt alone. She *was* alone. But their gesture comforted her.

But even in death, our benevolent guardian angel Lillian transformed our lives yet again.

CHAPTER 16

THE INHERITANCE

MOM NEVER PAID ANY ATTENTION WHEN AUNT LILLIAN WOULD SAY, "I'M remembering you in my will."

"At last, I'll have enough money to elope!" she joked.

So, it was a shock to learn that Lillian had indeed left her money. More than $30,000.

Dad likely expected her to hand it over and defer to his decisions, but she had other ideas. For the first time since they married, Mom had her own money. And we all had obvious needs. We girls were all in Catholic schools and wore uniforms, but Seamus and Tim attended Campus School, a privately operated but publicly funded school. They needed proper clothes. Mom went into a men's clothing store a block away and ordered such an extensive wardrobe that the owner delivered the order personally, stacking cardboard boxes in the living room filled with shirts, pants, socks, and ties.

Mom waited until Ellen had a good day, when her energy levels were a little higher than usual, and took us both downtown.

We wove through the crowded aisles of AM&As—then a fixture of Buffalo's bustling downtown—until we reached the section with the bedspreads. Mom picked one with a pattern covered in flowers and gave us a choice between two colors—pink or yellow. Ellen grabbed the yellow one immediately. I was left with the pink one, to my dismay. But having a bedspread at all was a novelty.

Then Mom began to furnish the house. Our furniture had become dilapidated from the pummeling of six children. She bought a large round oak table with lion's feet for the kitchen to replace the worn picnic table. We attended estate sales with musty rooms and hopeful prices, crowded with Empire couches, overstuffed wing chairs, and seemingly endless tables covered in crystal and silver of once-prominent Buffalo families. Mom had the hallway wallpapered, and the kitchen floor and front hallway tiled. She bought a dishwasher, an oriental rug, and a Scott record player and sound system to play her beloved classical music. At one point, we had more than a dozen antique couches.

When Christmas came, she bought us so many presents that she ran out of wrapping paper, and just piled them in stacks on the floor with name tags and the occasional ribbon.

But, beyond meeting our needs, Mom didn't really have a financial vision. That changed when Eugene Bangs called with an idea.

Gene Bangs owned a furniture store in Buffalo. Dad did business with him through his disaster services budget, which paid the store to provide furniture for families recovering from house fires. Gene also owned a restaurant, but he and his wife had tired of the demands.

They found a buyer for the restaurant, but he was short on cash, so he wheedled his wife into handing over the deed to a house she owned on East Cliff Island. The couple offered Gene the property to help close the deal.

Soon after, Gene asked my mother if she wanted to buy the house. Mom instantly agreed and paid $8,000. The house had two stories and new roof, and had recently been painted white. It had enough land for touch football games (and no need to stop for traffic, due to the lack of cars on the island). A large sunporch faced the harbor with its dancing sailboats and a dock where Ellen and I could continue in our quest to catch elusive sunfish.

While preparing paperwork, the lawyer asked whose names would be on the deed.

My father replied immediately. "Both of our names, of course."

"Absolutely not," Mom countered. "My money, my cottage."

Dad was shocked, but she didn't budge. The cottage would be in her name and became her place of refuge. And Ellen, when she was well enough, could get far away from the needles and the tests and hospital stays that were dominating her life.

The Island was about forty miles away. If Mom wanted to have easy access throughout the year to so remote a place, she had to figure out how to get there. At forty-six, Mom still hadn't learned to drive, so she arranged for lessons, then bought a used station wagon. She was ready for an adventure.

The first time she made the trip, she was visibly nervous. As she inched out of our driveway, she turned slowly onto Anderson Place as if piloting an ocean liner. I thought it would take her the entire day to make the drive, but after an hour she called us long distance from the Spinnaker.

"Maura, I made it!" she exulted, as if she had wended through the Bermuda Triangle and landed, unscathed.

It took me years to appreciate the true nature of her journey. Mom had not merely completed a trip of several dozen miles, navigating the highways of Buffalo and the rural, two-lane county roads beyond. The passage was transformative, from a life hemmed in by motherhood and matrimony and an inability to go anywhere that wasn't reachable by foot or by bus without my father's help or approval, to a greater freedom and a broader vision for her life.

Mom had a car, a bank account, and a house on the water that she dubbed "Toad Hall," after Mr. Toad's manse in the *Wind in the Willows*. She even purchased *The Banana Boat* from the Marins.

The money, of course, was finite. There were no investments to spin off more income. The balance on her newfound bank account inevitably dwindled. Dad never gave up control over paying the household expenses or his paycheck, but asked her for money "to pay bills" so frequently that she began to ask for the bills to pay them directly. He continued to lurch home long after we had gone to bed.

And Ellen was making no real progress toward regaining her health.

Yet, the cottage liberated all of us. We were no longer stuck in the city, with its worries, noise, and traffic. We had a place to go where the only sounds were that of waves crashing on the rocky shore. In May, we could watch the large ice floes from winter on the Great Lakes float by on Lake Ontario, making their annual journey toward the St. Lawrence River and out to sea. We could pack for the Island the moment school ended in June and stay until school began in September. When Ellen wasn't in the hospital, she and I could fish from our own dock. We could spend autumn weekends scuffing leaves from the towering silver maple trees that surrounded the house, when little could be heard but the honking of geese flying south.

CHAPTER 17

DODDERING ON THE LAKE

THE PREVIOUS OWNER INSISTED ON REMOVING EVERY STICK OF FURNITURE FROM the cottage. This was a radical departure from Island norms, where houses were traditionally sold with contents intact because it was highly laborious to move furniture off or onto the Island. Usually, if furniture was to be removed, the house was sold during the winter, when chairs and couches could be slid on sleds across the ice-covered harbor. When Island homes sold in warm weather, sellers included furnishings along with the keys.

Yet, Mrs. Hinkle would leave nothing behind.

That was fine by Mom. She was deeply sympathetic. Mrs. Hinkle had sacrificed a summer place she loved so her husband could chase a dream. And, in any event, the antiques were beginning to pile up in the house on Anderson Place, where we now had thirteen couches. The cottage's broad screened-in sunporch, with its large windows that opened like doors, was big enough for three couches. The living room could hold two.

The bedrooms of the cottage had the basics, but the rest of the house was bare. Dad assured my mother that he would oversee the precarious task of moving the furniture onto *The Banana Boat*, unloading and carting couches and chairs up twenty-seven stairs and into the house. Mom told me to take the rowboat and meet my father and brother Tim at the Spinnaker dock, where Dad had tied up *The Banana Boat* the night before. As I turned to go, Mom said, "For God's sake, tell your father I said not to overload the boat."

When I arrived, I could see the furniture truck that the Bangs lent us parked nearby, with no sign of activity.

Dad was in the bar drinking Labatts.

"Mom says not to overload the boat."

"She has no faith in me," Dad replied. "Have a 7-Up while I think through our strategy."

In a matter of seconds, he decided he could bring everything across the water in one trip.

I was doubtful. Despite *The Banana Boat* being seventeen feet long and broad in the beam, the truck was overflowing with couches, chairs, a kitchen table, and wicker furniture.

"Just one more beer," Dad said.

He downed the draft, then he and Tim began to make trips between the dock and the parking lot, shouldering the furniture and putting the heaviest couches on the bottom of the broad wooden boat. The abnormal sight drew a crowd in the Spinnaker's screened-in porch extending over the dock. Spectators ordered rounds of drinks and began to place bets on whether the furniture would make it to the island unscathed. Ruthie, the waitress, scurried between the bar and the porch, filling pitchers of beer and lining up shots for the growing crowd of onlookers.

Dad insisted on stacking the furniture like matchsticks, lighter items teetering on the heavier furniture that made up the foundation. Chairs and table legs interlocked in a way that made the whole thing almost look stable. One of the small Victorian fainting couches, destined for the porch, tilted precariously on the bow. The ever-enlarging crowd on the Spinnaker porch erupted in howls of laughter as Tim and Dad piled the furniture ever higher.

Then Dad stepped off *The Banana Boat* just as Tim put one foot on the gunwale, reaching over to balance one last item.

Dad heaved himself off the boat and stepped on the dock. *The Banana Boat* teetered. Tim did a perfect split, with one foot on the dock and one foot on the rapidly receding vessel. Like a cartoon character, he defied gravity for a few seconds, flailing, suspended between land and the eelgrass-choked water of the harbor below. He had time to curse before plunging in, rocking the drifting boat even more. After swaying for a moment, the fainting couch, the wicker furniture, and various other items tumbled down, plopping in the harbor waters around Tim like cannonballs. The Spinnaker crowd erupted in cheers and shrieks, with moans from those who lost wagers and hoots of triumph from those who won. A few onlookers hurried to help fish out the furniture—and Tim.

When Mom saw the overloaded, canary-colored boat come chugging across the harbor carrying a mountain of dripping furniture, she was irritated, but unsurprised.

"A little water never hurt anything," Dad said, when they finally reached the dock. "How about a cold beer?"

When the fainting couch finally dried out, it became my bed most nights. I rarely slept upstairs in my small, stuffy bedroom. I would fall asleep there, on the sunporch, listening to the rhythmic thrum of bullfrogs and the rustle of reeds.

Fishing, swimming, roaming, and reading were major forms of entertainment, along with visiting with neighbors, aided by another Island tradition. When people had not only arrived for the season, but were available and willing for others to pay a call, they would hang an American flag. If they were busy, preferring no visitors that day, they would put the flag in the house. What strangers might mistake for patriotism was code.

My search for the perfect next-door neighbor, with a girl my age to play with, was never fulfilled on the Island. It was virtually devoid of children. So many residents were elderly or near retirement that my mother's nickname for the place was "Doddering on the Lake." Yet, having grown up without grandparents, I didn't mind listening to stories of the elderly, and they in turn were endlessly patient with my questions.

Our neighbors on one side were a graying captain on the Buffalo police force and his wife. Their house, once the Island's only store and tavern, still had the trappings of its former life: a long mahogany bar; a huge, ornate, brass mechanical cash register; an old pinball machine; and a red-and-white cooler for Coca-Colas. The couple served us with elaborate ceremony whenever we visited.

Our neighbor on the other side was Bess Crawley, eighty and newly widowed. She had been spending summers on the island since she first arrived as a bride of twenty-six. Despite being wiry and small, as summer waned and the days began to cool I would regularly wake to the sound of her chopping kindling for her woodstove.

The cottage beside Mrs. Crawley was the home of Grace Cohen, her best friend and even older at eighty-five. Nearly six feet tall, Mrs. Cohen liked to sunbathe nude on her front lawn, stretching out with dish towels covering what she laughed were her "unmentionables." She was famous for her Jello, made with wine instead of water.

Down the sidewalk lived Irena, a member of the Buffalo Philharmonic who had survived the horrors of war-torn Eastern Europe and Nazi rule during the 1940s. She buried bad memories under constant construction, the sound of her hammering drywall or sawing lumber floating out from within her cottage at all hours.

Across the way was the elegant Margaret McMann, who had first come to the Island in 1912 at the age of fourteen when her family bought her cottage. Yet I learned to be especially vigilant around her husband Charlie, who would smirk as he served me lemonade. More than once, it was spiked with gin. Mrs. McMann taught me, by example, that small talk need never be trivial. Her attentive questions and comments made me feel welcome, even as her husband tried to ply me with booze.

Alcohol, in fact, was as much a part of Island life as flying the flag to attract company, the sight of the waves, or the constant reminder that the summer days were fleeting, and that the cool breath of autumn would soon arrive.

CHAPTER 18

BOOZE, THE CENTER OF LIFE

THE PEACE OF THE ISLAND AND THE TURMOIL OF THE CITY WERE CONNECTED BY one thing—the preponderance of alcohol. With its proximity to Canada, the Island became popular during Prohibition, and neighbors still swapped stories about its swashbuckling past. Stories abounded of rumrunners from the Island speeding across Lake Ontario to Canada and back, carrying crates of liquor to thirsty Americans. Many cottages, including ours, had secret compartments intended to hide alcohol. My bedroom floor had adjacent boards that opened like a book to reveal the space within. Some Islanders installed beer taps in their living rooms, with kegs transported from the docks to the top of the Island by determined residents. Most neighbors had one refrigerator for milk and groceries, and another for cases of beer.

Drinking was a daily ritual. Without streets or cars, there was no possibility of drunk driving. My parents kept a full liquor cabinet at the Island and trips to the town grocery store often included purchasing cases of "pounders," sixteen-ounce bottles of Genesee Cream Ale.

Alcohol, to me, was an object of both fear and attraction. It bestowed upon its users gaiety and celebration, relaxation, and revelry. While it had the power to uplift, it could also destroy. So much the former if the drinker could "hold his liquor" and not allow the substance to control him.

Drinking was my family's Olympic sport—the main social activity of an adult society I longed to join—and was intertwined with our pride in being Irish. I knew all the Irish drinking songs—a few from records of Tommy Makem and the Clancy Brothers, others derisively sung by my mother:

"The doors swing in/The doors swing out/
Some pass in/And others pass out!"
"Whiskey, you're the devil, you're leading me astray."

It was impossible to imagine St. Patrick's Day without raising a glass or three.

The Irish had a teetotaling tradition, too, that of "taking the pledge" not to drink as an adult. Dad's grandmother had taken the pledge and had been a committed non-drinker. Yet, during the 1960s in America, including within our family, choosing to abstain from alcohol was akin to madness—even if the true insanity arrived in bottles of rye whiskey, cases of beer, and an afternoon binge.

Adult beverages fueled good times and comforted in times of trouble. They made days brighter and conversation more amusing. People who didn't drink were either boring or religious extremists. Alcohol was the Dr. Feelgood elixir for just about anything that ailed. My brother Seamus unwittingly articulated this view when he was about ten years old and made up a rhyme, much to my parents' amusement: "*If you're cranky, take a tranky. If you're not, take a shot.*"

Alcohol was wonderful—until it wasn't. Fueling angry words, grief, and misunderstanding, it was poison, and yet, still, beloved. As a child I blamed my father for his behavior when he was drunk, but never the substance itself. Alcohol was too high on our family's unspoken hierarchy of values, too cherished to be the source of our problems. We blamed Dad for his moral shortcoming of over-indulging. None of us could understand why he didn't cut back. We knew little beyond newspaper advice columns about theories of addiction. They seemed ridiculous anyway, since nobody was forced to drink. The idea that addiction could develop one shot at a time, becoming a ruinous compulsion years before physical dependence, was beyond our understanding. Moreover, Dad didn't fit the profile of the alcoholic who pours a drink in the morning. His hands never shook from withdrawal after a bender. Dad got hangovers, but he almost never missed work because of drinking. He roared his anger and barely concealed his bitterness at home, but was hugely popular outside of it.

"He's a saint in the street, and a *divil* in the house," my mother would say, mimicking an Irish brogue. Occasionally, she told him he was an alcoholic and asked him to get help.

Dad refused, but he also latched onto the very concept of being an alcoholic as a handy excuse when he felt defensive the day after drunken scenes.

"I drink because I like the taste of the stuff," he would say. "The affect has nothing to do with it."

Other times he would say, "Your mother is right. I am an alcoholic. That's why I can't help but drink."

The implication was that negative consequences were just going to happen from time to time. Yet, his alcoholic status meant that he deserved sympathy, not recrimination. He was a victim. We should neither intervene nor blame him for what happened during bouts of over drinking. The insight that he was an alcoholic, and therefore sick, didn't result in the logical next step—that he *should* get help.

This became apparent when the Marins, our friends who introduced us to the Island and sold us *The Banana Boat*, showed up on the Island for a visit. Tom, Dad's old drinking buddy, was transformed. He was tanned, clear-eyed, and had lost weight. His wife seemed happy. Tom explained that he had given up drinking and regularly attended Alcoholics Anonymous meetings. His wife went to Al-Anon meetings to better understand what the years of his drinking had done to their family life. Tom said that there was more to life than drinking, and sobriety was a joyous and satisfying alternative.

Dad's hair nearly stood on end. I thought for a moment that he would thrust a crucifix in front of Tom's face as though he were a vampire. My father couldn't get him out of the cottage quickly enough.

"Good for Tom for realizing he couldn't handle it," Dad said later, pouring a beer. "That doesn't mean I can't hold my booze."

Dad was defensive about his drinking, but the truth was, alcohol had become the ninth, most beloved, and surely one of the most important members of our family.

Moreover, I couldn't wait until I was old enough to partake myself, my curiosity sparked by occasional sips of the Wild Irish Rose wine my parents kept in the refrigerator, and the warm feeling it made going down my throat. I wondered about beer, too, and could not wait to be able to have a full glass of my own. That would come far sooner than the legal drinking age of eighteen. Although, it would be years before I appreciated why Bacchus was both the god of alcohol, and of madness.

When Dad began drinking, tension rose. It was only a matter of time before an argument broke out. Eventually, Dad would leave, slamming the door.

Yet, our mother drank, too. Whiskey was her drug of choice, with ice, a little water, and a splash of ginger ale. Most of the time Mom drank socially with others who were drinking just as much. When she was alone and imbibed, however, a pall fell over her that was very different from my father's boozing.

Getting drunk never sparked my mother's rage. She didn't start fights over imagined slights or thwarted ambition. Instead, when she drank alone, my mother would brood, playing solitaire over and over while she silently mulled over an issue or the nature of life itself, often while listening to Jean Sibelius's violin concerto. When I walked into the house on Anderson Place and heard the notes of that weeping violin, I felt an urge to flee. The sounds of ice rattling in a glass and the Finnish composer's Concerto in D major usually meant that Mom was not only drinking, but depressed. It occurred often enough that I became hyper-vigilant for the signs that my strong, funny, and optimistic mother was tumbling, at least temporarily, into darkness.

The drunken, ugly scenes were mostly relegated to the city. The cottage was indisputably Mom's turf. Mom moved there in early summer and stayed through most of the warm months, depending on whether Ellen was out of the hospital.

By the time Mom bought the cottage, my older siblings had jobs and stayed in the city most of the summer. Claudia had allergies and the cottage gave her headaches, so she avoided it. Dad came to the Island on weekends, but less regularly as time went on. He had to work. He also could keep whatever hours or company he chose in the city, and my mother wasn't around to ask questions.

On the dwindling occasions where he accompanied us to the cottage, Dad would sometimes drive me back to the city. He used to keep in the car a bottle of a thick, white liquid antacid called Maalox, which he habitually gulped as he drove to quell the pangs from what he said was an ulcer.

My mother would have none of it.

"You don't have an ulcer, Casey, for Christ's sake," she would say. "You drink too much."

"The hell I do," he would insist. "It's an ulcer."

One day as he and I drove back from the cottage he began to complain about my mother and her many faults, his resentments on repeat.

"She is a terrible housekeeper," he said. She didn't pay enough attention to the family. She wasn't supportive enough of him. These diatribes always upset and befuddled me. Argue back and I'd be in trouble. Stay silent and I would be disloyal to my mother. Worse, he might think I agreed with him. The knot in my stomach tightened.

In the middle of his rant, Dad asked me to hand him the Maalox.

"It's on the floor near your feet."

I picked up the sturdy brown bottle, shook it briefly, opened the cap, and handed it to him.

My father, with his eyes on the winding country road, didn't notice that the cap was off. He began to shake the container as vigorously as usual. A thick, white liquid geyser erupted from the bottle, splattering against the car ceiling, the door, the windows, and dribbling all over my father.

"What the hell did you do?" he sputtered.

In the face of his rage, it was all I could do not to shriek with laughter as the chalky liquid dribbled from his hair, forming a thick, white coating on his face, arms, and draped over his chest like a shawl.

"Dad, I was just trying to *help*," I said, poker-faced, as I handed him a cloth to wipe the Maalox out of his eyes. He stopped complaining about Mom, at least for that afternoon.

Driving from the city to the cottage with Dad, particularly after sunset, had its own terrors. One of the country roads took us over the Niagara escarpment, the prominent, cliff-like formation most famous for Niagara Falls, which roared over its bank. The escarpment is hundreds of miles long, beginning in Wisconsin, threading through Canada, and twisting its way through Western New York. On the way to Newcott, most roads curved around the escarpment to make the climb up or down easier on automobiles and reduce accidents on slippery roads in winter.

All but one country lane, that is.

The road took us to the edge of the escarpment and slanted straight down, so steep it made our ears pop. The sudden drop-off made it seem as though the car was careening over the edge of the Earth. That road, of course, was the one that Dad preferred, particularly at night, when he had several kids in the car. Moonless nights were jet black, with little but the glimmer of distant farmhouses and the car's headlights to illuminate the crumbling, two-lane road ahead. Just as we were about to drive over the peak of the hill, Dad would turn off the headlights. We would scream in genuine terror. Dad would laugh, and seconds felt like hours while he continued to accelerate downward through the darkness. Then he would flick the lights back on, sometimes having to swerve from the ditches that lined the road.

It was heart-stopping, much like the rest of life with him.

His frequent absences from the cottage reduced the tension in our lives and made the Island even more of a refuge, both from him and the city.

Our neighborhood in the city was far safer than the projects, but it wasn't a refuge from rising crime across the city. One day thieves broke into our home and stole the expensive Scott sound system of which my mother was so proud, on which she loved to play classical music. Mom mourned its loss and replaced it with a cheap record player.

The city held terrors for our animals, too. One day in the house on Anderson Place, while petting the long fur of my beloved gray cat Tom, I felt a sticky patch. I looked down to see his blood covering my hand. Little Tom had a long slice on his right thigh. Someone had deliberately cut him, the veterinarian said, as he sewed him up. The incident frightened me. Bad enough that now—coupled with my fear of the tiny cat getting run over by a car—I worried that a random sadist would hurt him again. I breathed easier when we brought him with us to the Island for the summer.

It was the safest place I knew. I could, if I wished, wander outside at night in my pajamas. Nobody cared. Neighbors were kind. Dad stayed away.

The difficulties returned when the summer was over and we closed the cottage, emptying the refrigerator and draining water from pipes to keep them from freezing during winter. I would remove the screens from the sunporch, my unofficial bedroom. We would haul *The Banana Boat* onto higher ground and turn it over to shield it from the winter snow. Like squirrels gathering acorns before winter, our neighbors had their own end-of-summer routines. Everyone removed the flags that invited visitors in for conversation, rolling them up so they could be unfurled once again the following year.

We would wave goodbye to Mrs. Crawley, watching as she scurried back and forth across the harbor in her dinghy, loading up her car as she prepared to travel to Florida for the winter. I would make breakfast for Mom, my daily habit, then I would walk to my favorite beach to sit on a bleached log and write in one of my notebooks. Finally, we would lock the doors that had been open all summer, scuffing leaves on our way out. The city awaited, with its noise, turmoil, and tension.

CHAPTER 19

STARVING FOR SURVIVAL

LITTLE BY LITTLE, ELLEN'S UNRELENTING ILLNESS WORSENED AS HER KIDNEYS LOST function and impurities spilled into her bloodstream.

When I brooded about Dr. Hardy's voodoo-like curse—his medical prognosis that Ellen would never live to the age of eighteen—I told myself he was just plain wrong. But some days I was overcome by worry. Battling dark thoughts became harder, like shutting your eyes and ears in the middle of a thunderstorm: My denials didn't make the storm go away. Reality became hard to avoid.

Her disease was a day-to-day ordeal. Everyone involved was playing for time, hoping there would be some breakthrough, a miracle drug or new procedure that would increase the odds of Ellen's long-term survival. As Mary Hawking, one of her physicians, told me decades later, the perennial question medical staff discussed at meetings was simple: "Can we give Ellen one more summer?"

Science had so few weapons with which to fight the disease. One of the main treatments amounted to a delicate dance between starvation and death. Less food meant that less poison in the form of uremia would swirl in Ellen's body. She could have food only in tiny amounts. Protein was restricted to an ounce and a half of meat every other day. On the days when she did not have meat, she could eat one precious egg.

Ellen also had to avoid liquid, especially certain kinds. Milk and orange juice were off the table; too much potassium. Mostly, she only drank water, limited to 16–20 ounces—a little over a pint a day. Constant thirst was torture. Tomatoes, bananas, and avocados also were forbidden. Ellen adored watermelon, but eating the water-filled fruit was relegated to her daydreams.

She had to take more than a dozen pills each day to treat the disease and its side effects. Ellen hated to use up what she was allowed to drink only to accommodate her bitter-tasting medications, so she taught herself to gag down the pills using mere drops of water.

She grew ever thinner. The girl who once burst into a room now drifted listlessly, exhausted and anemic. Most often, she stayed on the living room couch. Now, with her energy limited, Ellen read more than she had before, finding solace in books that took her mind off the way she felt. The school district sent tutors to help her catch up with the schoolwork her hospitalizations disrupted. She leaned over her notebooks, her gaunt face and pale forehead furrowed in a slight frown as she concentrated. Her shoulders were so bony that they looked pointed even through her shirt, like the ends of a hanger holding a too-small sweater.

Helpless to aid her, yet increasingly jealous of the attention she received, I felt increasing resentment toward Ellen.

And I hated myself for it.

* * *

As much as everyone worried about Ellen and her illness hung over the household, we were rarely so upset that we could not eat. Our meals were basic and cheap. We ate spaghetti made with jars of tomato sauce, the occasional meatloaf or hamburgers, fish sticks, canned vegetables, tacos, rice dishes using canned chow mein, and my favorite, egg noodles and gravy. Potatoes—boiled, baked, mashed—were fit into as many meals as possible. In the summer, our diet improved as my mother made big salads with vegetables from roadside stands topped with my mother's home-made salad dressing.

Steak was a rarity. There were simply too many of us to serve it for dinner. But my parents wanted to make Ellen's tiny allotments of meat special, so my father began to purchase and prepare small chunks of steak for her to eat regardless of what the rest of us were having.

The tantalizing aroma of beef that Dad cooked for Ellen got to me. And seeing him carefully slice her piece—roughly two inches square—made my mouth water. I wanted some, too. I knew it wasn't allowed. Yet I couldn't resist asking.

"Can I have some?" I said, as he picked up the rare steak and placed it on Ellen's plate. Ellen looked at me, wordlessly.

"No," Dad said, handing the plate to Ellen.

"Why not?" I fumed.

"Because Ellen has a kidney condition," my father said, quietly.

Ellen stared at me, eyes large in her thin face, and then began to slice the meat in tiny pieces.

My feelings were unreasonable, I knew. Ellen would have gladly given me her tiny dinner in exchange for my healthy body even for a little while. I, on the other hand, would not switch places with her for any price. But rage and rational thought warred within me. The steak, sizzling and pink, was more tease than reality. She would eat it as slowly as she could, and afterwards still be hungry, starving even, while the rest of us gulped down glasses of powdered milk and stuffed ourselves with starches and lesser meats. We would push away from the table feeling full, something Ellen barely remembered from her recent past.

Ellen, shrunken in her chair, ate with us despite the contrast between her reality and ours, feebly grateful to be home from the hospital. Yet, anger and shame ate at me like termites.

The only other family we knew with a critically ill child handled the crisis very differently. The Samsons had four children. Like us, they had escaped the projects, but moved to the suburbs. Doctors diagnosed their teenage daughter with cancer around the same time Ellen became ill with kidney disease. She, too, went in and out of the hospital, but not Children's Hospital like Ellen. Instead, she was often admitted for treatment to Roswell Park, the famous cancer treatment center in downtown Buffalo. Amidst the family uproar of trying to cope with a teenager's chronic illness, her mother enrolled everyone in therapy—group, family, and individual. They needed help to handle the stress, she told us, sitting in our kitchen one day.

My mother was aghast. She could not imagine airing family laundry to total strangers—in group therapy, no less! Her reaction ranged from disbelief to a mildly patronizing attitude.

"Well," she would say. "You do what you have to do to manage, I guess. We aren't there yet."

Taking my cue from Mom, I assumed that we didn't need the intervention of counselors, psychologists, and social workers. We had each other. Most of all, we had our sense of humor, which sharpened by the day. Our anger and fear distilled into sarcasm. Humor kept us from bursting into tears.

Still, sparks of unreasoning resentment burned within me no matter how I tried to push them away. Steak envy was the least of it. I had more and more problems at school, and Ellen could neither protect me nor keep me company. Tongue-tied around my peers, clueless about the latest rock music, quiet and constantly worried about Ellen, I had no friends. Yet, no one asked how I was doing. Ellen had become the dark star around which the family revolved. If she had a good day, so would we. If she was in crisis, we were plunged into the maelstrom right along with her.

But we couldn't talk about it. Complete honesty was off the table. Silence was the unspoken, unwritten rule, as if we had all taken vows against discussing the issues in any prolonged, serious way. Sure, we could joke about this slow-moving, unending crisis. We—especially Ellen—could make wisecracks about the hospital, the doctors, the ever-mounting number of pills she took every day. But otherwise, we avoided the topic altogether—even with each other.

Instead, she and I pretended.

* * *

We shared our daydreams in a setting far away from adults: A deserted, stony beach at the end of the Island where we would make a driftwood fire and talk about how, someday, everything would be different.

There would be no more needles, pills, or pain. Ellen could eat as much watermelon as she wanted. She dreamt of her first full meal: mashed potatoes and gravy; sliced, fat tomatoes, crusty with salt and sprinkled with basil; thick slabs of steak or roast turkey;

full glasses of ice-cold whole milk. She wanted, most of all, to have her energy back. Maybe she would even join an athletic team. Ellen longed to row with a crew team like our brothers.

I pointed out that the West Side Rowing Club had never allowed women to join the sport.

"But the Canadian crew teams have women," Ellen would say. We had seen them the last time we went to St. Catharines, Ontario, to watch the boys race.

"Well, then, maybe," I would say, poking at the fire.

One night, within the comforting shelter of leaning willow trees, we fed chunks of wood slowly into the flames and I cooked a thin soup, cutting up potatoes and beef bouillon and settling a small pan over the coals. Ellen took a tiny sip and shook her head.

"Too salty for me. But someday, when I am not sick, we will come here, and I will have as much as I want."

"Let's swear on it," I said.

We pricked our thumbs to draw a drop of blood. I winced as Ellen smirked. "This is nothing," she said.

We rubbed our thumbs together.

"Now we have to do it," Ellen said. "No matter how long it takes, we have to come here when I'm not sick anymore."

"Now you *have* to get better."

I told her nothing of the burden of knowledge I carried. My mother and I never discussed the awful day Mom had blurted out the doctor's grim prophesy to ten-year-old me. I never told anyone.

I decided the prognosis was a mistake. Against all odds, Ellen would prove just how wrong he was. She would get through the gauntlet of needles and pills, hospital stays, the hunger and thirst, the anemia and bone-weariness, and make it back to the beach for as much soup as she wanted, no matter how salty.

CHAPTER 20

DIALYSIS

BESIDES EATING AND DRINKING NEXT TO NOTHING, MEDICAL SCIENCE HAD ONE major tool to keep Ellen alive: dialysis. At first, she received hospital-based peritoneal dialysis to ease the strain on her kidneys. This involved the insertion of a tube into her abdominal cavity, through which flowed fluid made up of glucose, sodium, chloride, calcium, and other minerals. The liquid absorbed salt and other elements her kidneys could no longer remove. Afterward, nurses drained the waste-filled fluid from her abdomen. Ellen, and her struggling kidneys, were then ready to fight on.

After nine months or so of this procedure, it was clear that thirteen-year-old Ellen needed dialysis regularly. That meant that she had to go on hemodialysis; two to three times a week she would be hooked up through her arm to a large machine that would filter her blood and remove waste, doing the job that her kidneys could not. The reason patients, including Ellen, could get regular hemodialysis was because of a new surgical technique developed in 1966 to keep their veins healthy.

Doctors performed surgery on Ellen's arm to connect an artery and a vein under the skin of her right wrist. After healing, the vein grew larger and walls thicker with increased blood flowing from the artery, providing easy access to insert the large needles from the dialysis machine into Ellen's right arm (she was left-handed) and helped speed the flow of blood through the machine's filters.

"Come feel this," she said to me after the surgery.

I touched her arm and jumped back. The blood surged through a swollen vein slightly raised in her arm. The vein was engorged with blood, like rapids surging below her skin.

Ellen laughed.

"It feels like electricity," I said.

I got a buzzing sensation when I touched her arm. This delighted Ellen. She loved to freak people out by daring them to touch her wrist and watching them react the same way I did.

Twice a week, eight to ten hours at a time, hemodialysis machines would act as Ellen's kidneys, giving her a little more freedom. She could be treated at an outpatient clinic for the procedure. When I didn't have school I could go with her, since the clinic allowed visitors under the age of fourteen. I didn't have to stand outside in the hospital parking lot, peering at her distant face in a window as we waved at one another. But each time hemodialysis began, Ellen and the nurses asked me to step out while they attached her to the machines. The needles were the size of construction nails and insertion was always painful.

Ellen rarely mentioned it.

Once she was connected, I could stay by her side all day. We could play rummy and talk. Sometimes we would read books in companionable silence. Yet other days her headaches debilitated her. She would feel cold or experience muscle cramps. From time to time, she would doze. To her delight, while she was on dialysis she could eat anything she wanted, as long she was attached to the churning machine.

It was existence. It prolonged her life. But to me, it wasn't really living.

The aftermath of dialysis for Ellen was usually fatigue and intractable nausea. No matter what momentary pleasure she experienced from eating a normal meal, it would often come up later. She didn't complain. If we were driving to the cottage—an hour-long trip—she would vomit quietly and continually in the plastic bags she always remembered to grab before leaving the clinic.

Despite having to return to her strict diet and her health still precarious after her treatments, there were glimmers of the old Ellen—the one so lively, so funny, and with such energy and spark.

On one particular autumn day, Claudia, Ellen, and I were sitting on the porch at Anderson place, when Claudia mentioned that our neighbor Ann, who lived across the street, had upset her years before for revealing our father's affair. Ellen, who didn't like the neighbor anyway, needed no encouragement to plot immediate revenge.

Ellen looked at Claudia, then across the street. We all knew that Ann, an executive secretary, came home at 6 p.m.—soon. Twilight was gathering.

Ellen turned to me.

"Got a penny?" She asked.

I fished a penny out of the pocket of my jeans and handed it to her.

Wordlessly, she stood up and walked across the street. I followed, curious.

Ann's apartment was on the first floor of the three-unit house. Her routine was the same, we knew, from witnessing it for years. She would open the front door, step in the small entryway inside, and turn on the light. Then she would unlock her apartment door, and turn on the lights in the living room, brightening the front picture window of the house.

Ellen unscrewed the lightbulb from the fixture on the wall that illuminated the entryway in front of the apartment door. She made sure the switch was off, then dropped the penny in the socket and screwed in the lightbulb once again.

"What are you doing?" I asked, confused.

"Just wait."

We went back to the porch and took our seats, ready for the show.

Ann arrived on time, parked her car, entered the house, then flicked on the light.

The light went on, then turned off. Immediately.

Ellen began to giggle. Claudia looked confused. I was curious.

We could see Ann in the gathering gloom flicking on and off the switch impotently. Then she went inside the apartment. She tried turning on lights in her living room and dining room. Nothing worked.

The easiest way to get in the basement of the house was through the side door. She stomped out, and went downstairs to change the fuses on the electrical panel.

She trudged back upstairs and turned on the hall light. Now all the lights in the apartment flashed on, and we could almost hear her sigh of relief.

Then, as the electrical short caused by the copper penny in the socket did its work, every light in her apartment went out again.

We all started to giggle.

Ann ran around to the side of the house, holding another fuse. She went downstairs to the basement again and repeated the process over and over.

Ellen began to howl with delight. She couldn't stop. Tears streamed down her face.

Claudia laughed, too, shaking her head. I looked at Ellen in wonderment. Even now, I have no idea how she figured out how to cause an electrical short that would disrupt the life of our gossipy neighbor and give us all a ringside seat to her well-deserved distress.

Mom called us in for dinner. We trooped into the house, giggling. The lights across the street went on and off repeatedly, like an SOS signal in the gathering darkness.

CHAPTER 21

"DEAD EYE! DEAD EYE!"

BEING CONFIRMED WAS ONE OF THE HIGH POINTS OF ATTENDING A CATHOLIC elementary school. But as Ellen's school attendance grew spottier due to her illness, her ability to stay out of the hospital long enough to experience this religious milestone became uncertain.

Nobody wanted her to miss it. Nuns told us that the sacrament of confirmation would make us "soldiers of Christ." It was the ceremony through which we took a new middle name (a saint's name, subject to clergy approval) and confirmed our belief in the One, True, Holy, Catholic, and Apostolic Church. We were taught that this was the completion of the journey we began at baptism and that it would seal our belief in Catholicism. In return, the Holy Spirit would shower graces upon us, as sort of a heavenly quid pro quo for our commitment to the religion of our birth.

The ritual was inevitable, hardly something we could refuse without risking family shame and social banishment. The idea that any elementary school student in our orbit would come to confirmation with a mature, questioning, and independent mind was absurd. Any glimmering of theological doubt was swept away in anticipation of pleasant family attention and cards with crisp dollar bills that aunts and uncles tucked inside.

Confirmation would be the highlight of sixth grade.

However, Ellen was too sick to be confirmed with her classmates the year they received the sacrament. The next year, she attended as many of the preparation sessions as she could with the other students, but the week of the ceremony, she was in the hospital. When Father Garvey heard that Ellen was unlikely to attend for a second year, he called the bishop of Buffalo, James McNulty. Bishop McNulty, to his credit and no doubt heeding the request of a friend and fellow Irishman, said if Ellen couldn't come to the church, the Church would come to her. He would confirm her in her hospital room, which, after all, was just a half block from the bishop's stately mansion.

McNulty entered the fifth floor of Children's Hospital glorious in flowing vestments, carrying a shepherd's crook and wearing a tall, gold-embroidered miter on his head. The bishop solemnly greeted our parents, took Ellen's hand, and talked to her quietly. After a few minutes he made the sign of the cross with chrism, consecrated oil on her forehead, and said, "Be sealed with the gift of the Holy Spirit," to which Ellen replied, "Amen." He left her a gift: A carved, Italian marble statue of the Virgin Mary holding baby Jesus. My mother was thrilled with the fine artistry of the intricate sculpture, and my father was impressed.

Surely, the Holy Spirit would bless Ellen and improve her health, we thought.

Soon thereafter, Ellen lost the ability to see out of her left eye.

It happened without warning. She might have had a spike in blood pressure that caused a blood clot in her retinal artery.

Medication couldn't always control Ellen's blood pressure, which was erratic due to her failing kidneys. This side effect, however, was new and unexpected.

The doctors hoped that her vision would come back eventually, but the eye began to increase the frequency and intensity of her headaches. Over time, it swelled up and developed a scarlet hue. Ellen tried to comb her hair over the distended orb in a futile attempt to keep people from noticing it. Not only was she thin from her strict diet, and thirsty, but she had a monstrous eye as she entered adolescence.

I soon learned that the eye was sensitive to the slightest touch.

One day, when I was twelve and Ellen fourteen, I was excited to attend an event with my sister Claudia at her high school. Ellen, in the third year of her illness, didn't feel well enough to go, so Claudia's friend Terry came with us. She was kind and easy to talk to, asking me serious questions about school, my interests, and how Ellen was doing. Before I left to ride home, Terry said to me, "Tell Ellen that we all hope she gets better. And give her this from me."

She leaned forward and gave me a kiss on the cheek.

Giddy from the unaccustomed attention, I entered the house happier than I had been in a long time. I approached Ellen, who was in the kitchen with Mom, and smiled.

"Terry told me to give you something," I said. I leaned forward and brushed aside her hair so I could give her a kiss on the cheek.

The back of my fingernails must have barely brushed the distended eyelid of her blind eye as I pushed aside her hair. Ellen's head jerked back, and she burst into tears.

I was horrified. My stoic sister never, ever cried.

Ellen quickly got control of her emotions, and wiped away her tears. "What did Terry want you to give me?"

"A kiss," I said miserably. "A kiss on the cheek."

I walked out of the kitchen, went to my room, and curled up on my bed, feeling like an ax murderer.

The eye so altered her looks that other students began to react, although Ellen's absenteeism and gang of friends shielded her from the worst.

Our school, like most, prohibited physical fights, but largely ignored verbal cruelty and teasing among children, particularly males teasing females.

Boys harassed me every day in school, too. My parents, always distracted by Ellen's ever-worsening health, told me to ignore the constant mockery and it would go away. I followed their advice, but the bullying only intensified. I didn't have the foggiest idea how to protect myself from the abuse.

However, when the same boys turned on Ellen while we walked home one day, I reacted with instant ferocity.

We must have left school later than usual, because we walked home alone, without the usual river of students. We crossed a busy street, where four boys were waiting.

One boy began to jeer.

"Dead eye! Dead eye! Look at the dead eye!"

He pointed at Ellen and laughed.

The others began to point and laugh, too. Then they surrounded us.

As I heard the taunts, I instantly became enraged and felt no fear at all. I was carrying two books, one of which I hurled at the ringleader, Jake, and ignored the other three circling around us. Startled, he ducked, but not fast enough. The book slammed on the side of his head. But I wasn't done.

As Ellen had so many years before when she protected me in second grade, I shouted, "Leave my sister alone, you jerk!"

I pounded him with my remaining book. It was our social studies textbook, always the thickest; I slammed it over his head several times, as fast and as hard as I could. Jake squealed and scrambled away. His friends forgot about my sister and me. Instead, Jake
became the target of their mockery. They walked down the street
laughing at him and left us alone.

I looked at Ellen, panting from the effort and the ferocity of my
rage. She looked at me with admiration and sadness. The protector
now had become the protected.

Ellen's terrible and exacting illness allowed all of us moments
of heroism.

Even my father.

Soon after the altercation with the boy, while we were all staying overnight at the cottage, Ellen rushed into our parents' room
sobbing hysterically at 3 a.m. She had for months not seen out
of her left eye. Now her right eye, her good eye, the eye that still
twinkled with occasional laughter and gave her the blessing of
superb eyesight, throbbed in pain ominously.

"I'm going blind! I'm going blind!" she wailed.

Dad jumped into his clothes and told Mom to call Children's
Hospital.

"We will be there in a half hour," he said. He grabbed Ellen,
flew down the stairs to the dock, and with a roar of *The Banana
Boat*, they were gone.

Dad barely stopped to tie up the boat at the Spinnaker
dock. Bundling Ellen in the car, he drove a hundred miles an
hour over quiet country roads, then highways, speeding toward
the hospital.

He covered forty miles in less than a half hour and one of the
doctors met them at the door of the emergency room.

Medical tests showed that Ellen's remaining good eye was not threatened. Her blood pressure was normal. She may have experienced a simple sinus headache.

Yet, after discussing the situation with Ellen and my parents, her physicians concluded that sight would never return in Ellen's left eye. Hoping that her vision would come back was no longer worth the pain it inflicted—not only physical, but psychological.

Doctors soon removed her eye. It was gone forever, replaced by one made of plastic.

CHAPTER 22

BULLIES AND PROTESTS

PRAYING FOR ELLEN OFFERED ME A FEW RAYS OF HOPE, ENCOURAGED BY WEEKLY Mass and prayers before classes began at school. The Catholic elementary school I attended two blocks from our home was an ecclesiastical factory subsidized by the Roman Catholic Diocese of Buffalo. The only cost to Catholic families for their children to attend was a small textbook rental fee for each child. The aim was to sow a crop of good Catholics for harvesting later in adulthood. Religious fealty was mandatory. We had to go to Mass every week or face the wrath of the nuns. Confession, later called the Sacrament of Reconciliation, was a monthly event in which each one of us would prepare to whisper our many shortcomings. I would line up with my fellow students and when my turn came, enter the darkness of a wooden room the size of a telephone booth. Kneeling, I would recite my sins to a bored priest who sat behind a screen.

But I wondered about the school's insistence on adhering to a schedule of religious ritual while ignoring acts that mattered. The school was a cesspool of loathsome adolescent behavior. Teasing and cruelty won the day. Kindness got lip service.

The principal of the school was meek Sister Leo, who was dark haired, dark eyed, emotional, proudly Italian, and about fifty. Every year, she suggested that Father Garvey give the students a half-day off for St. Joseph's feast day, March 19, not only the namesake of the school, but the patron saint of Sicily. Alas, the feast day was too close to St. Patrick's Day on March 17, Father Garvey's preferred saint and the one whose feast day he chose to honor every year by granting students time off to celebrate.

Sister Leo was accustomed to being ignored. She had so little control over students that once, unable to make the chaos in the cafeteria subside by shouting for silence, stamping her feet, and ever more insistently ringing a large brass bell that was supposed to call for order, she sat down and wept while students at the surrounding lunchroom tables became hysterical with laughter.

Once she hired Sister Hildegard to teach sixth grade, Sister Leo became downright inconsequential, and the pretense of modeling Christian values fell away entirely. While Sister Leo retained the title of head of school, for the next three years, Sister Hildegard, with her beet-red face, small blue eyes, and a German's love of order, ran the place like a summer camp for Hitler Youth.

Sister Hildegard rarely smiled. She was exacting about rules, no matter how trivial, and invented others on her own authority. And she had a mean streak.

She ruled by fear. She threatened pupils—boys and girls alike—with corporal punishment, which until then I had neither experienced nor witnessed in school. Early on in her tenure, she even carried out a vicious public paddling of one of the few Black students in the school in front of our classroom, which terrified us and enraged him. When she handed him the paddle to return to the principal's office and turned away, he raised it behind her head as if to hit her, and we all silently cheered him on. Of course, he didn't follow through—he didn't dare. He lowered the wooden weapon and walked away. The incident was humiliating, unnecessary, and designed to scare the hell out of us. We all cowered as one.

The ugly scene added to the predatory atmosphere. Sister Hildegard was a bully, her actions magnified because she had so much power. But students followed her example. Bullying became common. Interventions were rare. I was a regular target, and reacted with a humiliated and fearful silence.

Yet, when it came to standing up for others, I intervened immediately with a sense of injustice and a certainty I never felt on my own behalf. When boys targeted my ailing sister, I lashed out. But when adolescent bullies mocked me, I froze.

A handful of boys made up jokes about my hair, my looks, my teeth, my voice. They told me I was stupid. They warned others to stay away.

And they did.

Two in particular were my main tormenters. Jordan took the lead and Axel took the supporting role of laughing at whatever Jordan did. They pushed up their noses in imitation of my Irish turned-up nose and snorted like a pig. They talked, loudly, about how I smelled and held their noses. Other male classmates laughed at the abuse. A precious few neither laughed nor joined in, and I always felt grateful to them.

The girls, for the most part, avoided me. They wouldn't include me in the comforting groups of two and four walking to or from school, eating lunch together, or fixing their hair in the bathroom.

Perhaps they hoped to avoid the daily negative attention the boys heaped on me.

Going to school every day felt like entering a snake pit.

I wondered why I couldn't blend in.

For starters, other girls had a carefree manner that I envied but couldn't manage. Classmates ironed their locks so they were fashionably straight, while I left my long black hair in its natural state.

In class, when we were asked to write a paper on music we enjoyed, my fellow students extolled The Beatles, The Doors, The Monkees, and The Mamas and the Papas. Rock music was what the popular kids listened to, and was not my genre of choice, so I wrote a paper about the music of Mozart and Rachmaninoff and read it aloud to stunned silence.

Ellen's health was constantly on my mind, but I had learned not to talk about it. So, I stayed quiet nearly all the time. I was timid. Vulnerability attracts attention, usually the wrong kind.

Coming up with ways to make the boys stop teasing was challenging. If I went to teachers, the bullies would retaliate. Fighting every day was out of the question, and besides I was too small. When I went to my parents for help, they told me to ignore the insults, but that just fed the fire.

Compounding on the bullying and Ellen's health issues, the increasing turmoil of the 1960s seemed to reflect the agitation within our home, but for vastly different reasons. The country was like a clenched fist. Every day the headlines blared: A NATION TORN BY BOMBINGS AND RIOTS, DEMONSTRATIONS AGAINST THE VIETNAM WAR, and THE LONG OVERDUE CALL FOR CIVIL RIGHTS. Dr. Martin Luther King, Jr. dominated news stories every week, leading protests and calling for justice.

Then a white supremacist shot and killed Dr. King. Most adults I knew, including the school faculty, were deeply shaken. Yet, most were at a loss how to talk about it with students. Instead, we sang. In school, nuns herded all the students, overwhelmingly White, into the gym. They led us in singing every single verse of "We Shall Overcome."

We dimly grasped—in a purely intellectual way—some of the injustices foisted upon Black Americans. But we White children had no real idea what the words of the song really meant. And we had no idea what "we" would overcome in the haunting words of that song.

The school also decided around this time that the sixth, seventh, and eighth graders should see a movie dealing with the issues of justice. This was a radical decision. We students never got to see a movie in school.

Given events happening in the country, one would have thought that a movie such as *To Kill a Mockingbird* would have been appropriate, along with a conversation about what Black Americans had faced throughout American history. Inexplicably, the school chose to show us *The Phenix City Story*, a blood-soaked 1955 movie about intimidation, murder, and mayhem in Phenix, Alabama, that involved not segregation, but organized crime. The climax is an utterly terrifying scene in which the White, corrupt evil-doers throw the body of a murdered, ten-year-old Black girl onto the lawn of an anti-corruption crusader in full view of his screaming, hysterical children. A note pinned to the body says something to the effect of, "This will happen to your children, too."

The gruesome scene sent a ripple of terror through us, children who were not much older than the murdered girl in the movie. We

115

stared at each other, eyes wide with shock. Graphic violence continued on screen until the Army finally arrived and armored vehicles rumbled downtown in a muscular triumph of law and order. When the blood bath was over, the lights went on and we were all dismissed, traumatized, and to figure out what the hell the moral was supposed to be. When I blurted out to my mother after school that I had spent the afternoon watching this terrifying film, she asked, "They showed you kids *The Phenix City Story*? What in God's name were they thinking?"

What, indeed. But the lesson, to me, was this: In the midst of chaos in the country, in school, at home, and on the screen, those in power usually triumphed while those fighting for justice were squashed like bugs. I began questioning whether it helped anyone to push back or speak up.

But, once in a while, I did, in a very small way.

Indignation gave me a brief flash of courage when one of the more agreeable teachers got angry enough at the refusal of several boys to quiet down when she demanded classroom silence that she assigned the entire class homework as a form of punishment. We were all told to copy a chapter from our social studies book, and hand it in the next day. Most of the class was outraged that the disobedience of a few was to be paid for by the labors of the many, but we knew there was no choice.

Still, the situation enraged me. I looked at the chapter, which seemed endless, and instead, decided to write a letter objecting to the injustice of it all.

In the letter, I stated that I hadn't done anything, and that making me do this assignment was a blot against humanity. I consulted frequently with a dictionary and told my mother what I was doing. She thought my response was hilarious. When I stalled on wording, she helped me. I spent at least as much effort in writing the letter as I would have in completing the assignment. I signed it: "Indignantly and Maliciously Yours, Maura Casey."

The next day, the teacher demanded we all hand in the assignment, which every student but me had completed. She read my letter, stunned, and immediately told me to go out in the hallway.

Going in the hallway usually meant trouble. It was the elementary school equivalent of durance vile, of having committed a sin so grievous that we couldn't get yelled at in the classroom. My heart raced. I broke out into a cold sweat. I had never been sent to the hallway before. The teacher joined me after a few minutes and leaned against the wall to talk. In retrospect, she was probably amused. I found out, years later, that she and my mother were acquaintances, so she could probably guess who had come to my aid, and indeed egged me on. She didn't yell at me or threaten to call my parents. She told me not to do it again and we went back in the classroom.

But then Sister Hildegard heard about my nascent rebellion. She was not amused. A few days later, beet red, she burst in into our classroom, interrupting our teacher.

"You," she said, jabbing a fat forefinger in my direction. "Out in the hallway."

I froze, nearly wetting myself from terror. For a moment, I was paralyzed.

"Now," she snarled.

Somehow, I got up. Wobbly, I walked out of the classroom, closing the door behind me.

Then the harangue began. Sister Hildegard did not, as the young lay teacher had, lean against the wall to converse. No drill sergeant could have done a better job at an act of pure intimidation. She loomed over me, furious at my impertinence. She said I had insulted the teacher, the school, and my community. She said what I had done was a sin against God Himself and I had better remember it for confession. She raged and threatened me with expulsion. I shook and said nothing.

When she finished, she told me to go back in the classroom. I put my hand on the doorknob, trying my best not to dissolve into tears.

"Wait. One last thing," she said.

Now what? I thought.

"Who helped you write that letter?" she snapped, her piggy eyes narrowing. "Who had the nerve? And don't try to lie."

I realized she thought other students were in on the writing. This mystified me. *Those idiots?* I thought. I shook my head.

"Tell me," she said, her voice rising.

"It was my idea, but my mother helped. To tell you the truth, she helped a lot."

Sister Hildegard's eyes bulged in shock, and she stepped back.

"Your *mother* helped you?"

I nodded.

"Huh," she said. She was so completely caught off guard that she didn't know what to say. Finally, she told me to go back in the classroom and walked away.

My confession about my mother's involvement, with its implication that she was my ally, gave me something faintly resembling the upper hand. But I didn't know why—or how. All I knew was that I had escaped Sister Hildegard's clutches. I knew too well that it could be worse.

Later, I told my mother what had happened.

"You handed in that letter? Really? I thought the whole thing was a joke."

CHAPTER 23

AFTER-SCHOOL CHOICES

DURING THE SCHOOL DAY, I WAS ALWAYS HYPER-VIGILANT, WAITING FOR MOCK-ery or some other form of verbal abuse. But after school, I had choices.

Although I was often anxious when my father was at home, I liked that he worked for the Red Cross, with its sprawling campus of retrofitted mansions, three blocks from my elementary school. The place was kind and quirky. I stopped by after school once or twice a month, not to visit him, but because the organization was always on the lookout for volunteer help. There was always some task to do.

After saying hello to adults in different departments for an hour or two, I would file reports, stamp certificates for safety courses, or assemble gift bags of toiletries for shipment overseas to soldiers fighting in the Vietnam War. Dad was popular among his co-workers for his sense of humor and ability to recruit volunteers. I kept quiet about his behavior at home, and he never objected to me stopping by his work.

Once I finished my tasks, sometimes I would go to the Jewish Community Center across the street, which had excellent recreational facilities—a weight room, saunas and steam rooms, a gymnasium, a game room, and an indoor pool. Anyone was welcome to join, and everyone we knew did. Believers and atheists alike were members.

Normally, a family membership was a luxury costing hundreds of dollars every year, but not for us. My father had convinced his superiors to allow the JCC to use the Red Cross parking lot across the street. In return, the JCC gave him a free, lifetime membership for he and my mother. The center also gave us kids free memberships until we were twenty-one, in gratitude to our father.

Having access to indoor athletic facilities was a novelty for all of us, and I was at first startled to see naked bodies in the women's locker room. Modesty prevailed at home. With so many kids, we followed strict rules of privacy, knocking on anybody's bedroom door before entering. Men's bodies, of course, were mysteries. I had never seen an unclothed man.

Yet, in the JCC locker room, ladies walked around without a stitch of clothing, laughing and talking after swimming or sitting in the sauna. Some were thin; others were sashaying mountains of flesh. After the initial shock, locker-room nudity didn't bother me in the least. So when I planned to go to the Red Cross after school, besides carrying a bathing suit, I always made sure to remember to bring a small towel.

It never occurred to me that the towel could be used as a gag.

One day, in mid-October of 1969, I walked to my father's office after school, performed some small tasks, decided to skip the swim, and began to walk the five blocks home.

With two blocks to go, I had a choice: I could walk down the city sidewalks of West Utica, take a right on Atlantic Avenue, and a left on Anderson Place. Or I could save five minutes and walk through the abandoned half-block of trees and bushes that made up Dale's Lot.

Crumbling brick pillars on either side of a long driveway implied that the acreage was once the setting for a great home, like the Gilded-Age mansions that lined Delaware Avenue. Every mother in the neighborhood shooed us away from the area, and every kid in the neighborhood ignored the warnings. So many kids used its expanse as a shortcut to our neighborhood that a path had been worn down through the grass growing in the driveway.

Dale's Lot was a refuge from the sound of traffic that made up the discordant symphony of our lives. Once there, you could hear no traffic.

And those outside couldn't hear you scream.

CHAPTER 24

DALE'S LOT

As I VIEWED THE BUSHY CONFINES OF DALE'S LOT THAT AUTUMN AFTERNOON, I paused. I held my textbooks in one arm with their yellow book covers emblazoned with the bishop's coat of arms. On top was a towel, unused, since I hadn't swum. I wore a sweater. It had snowed earlier that month, but this afternoon was about sixty degrees, and evening promised to be fine. I was tired and felt a slight backache from carrying the books, so shaving off a few minutes of my commute was appealing.

The sun went behind the clouds and the wind grew colder. I shivered and felt a strong sense of foreboding. I stepped on the grassy space. *Don't do this*, I sensed. The feeling of dread grew. But everyone knew that feelings were irrational. I shrugged at the screaming sirens of my intuition and began walking through the weedy and overgrown grass.

Halfway through the lot, I saw a man out of the corner of my eye. He was to my left about fifty yards away, with black hair, dark eyes, pale skin, and a five o'clock shadow. He was slight of build and wearing a light jacket.

He covered the ground between us faster than I thought possible and grabbed me. I started to cry out, even as I knew there was no one to hear. He clapped his hand over my mouth and dragged me into the bushes.

"I'm not going to hurt you," he said, breathing heavily. My books scattered, yellow covers bright against red fall leaves strewn on the hard ground.

Then he saw the towel. He grabbed it and tightened it over my mouth.

"I'm not going to hurt you," he said again, pushing me down on the dirt.

He yanked up the skirt of my uniform as he unzipped his pants, pulled off my underwear, and crushingly, laid on top of me, humping desperately. He was heavy and sweating. I was terrified. What was he doing? He pushed and pushed. I wanted to struggle, yet I was pinned to the ground and frozen in fear.

The gag made me choke. I couldn't breathe. He was bigger than me and stronger. I was small and weak. I was nothing, not a person at all, just an inconsequential thing to be used and discarded. I knew in the core of my being that I didn't matter.

I was so alone.

After what seemed like an eternity of pushing, he got up, carefully cupping his hands around his penis. He turned away and zipped up his pants.

He loomed over me, gazing at the twelve-year-old whose life he had just shattered.

Then he smirked.

"See? I told you I wouldn't hurt you," he said.

He ran away.

I lay motionless for a few moments. Then I sat up. I untied the towel around my mouth and threw it away. It was striped, yellow, white, and black. I never wanted to see it again. I picked the leaves out of my hair and sweater. I found my underwear discarded under a bush and put it on, then gathered my scattered textbooks and stacked them in a pile.

There was nobody but me in Dale's Lot. Numbness washed over me.

The man had fled, but he could not have gotten far. He was probably just a block or two away. Maybe he was even passing by my house, where my mother, unsuspecting, was making dinner.

I stumbled out of the brushy acreage where, discarded in the leaves, lay the gag that I would spend years of my life untying.

CHAPTER 25

THE AFTERMATH

I BEGAN TO WALK HOME.

I managed not to cry until I collapsed inside the front hallway of our home, books scattering. I screamed that a man attacked me.

My cries sparked an instant uproar. Mom hugged me, then reached for the phone. Claudia put her arms around me. My mother called my father, her voice controlled.

"I'd like to speak with Mr. James Casey," she said, then, as the operator connected her to his office, she lowered her voice.

I could hear him almost wailing on the other end of the line.

"But she was just *here*!"

Then my mother called the police, who arrived in moments. Two officers interviewed me, then went to look for a man that I had described, which fit approximately half the males in the area. The policemen shook their heads as they left.

My mother took me to a hospital. Not Children's Hospital—so close by, so familiar that any one of us could have navigated its corridors blindfolded—but a hospital across the city, close to the projects we had left years before. The police told my mother that Meyer Memorial Hospital was equipped to do a careful exam.

The doctor who examined me was grave and serious, eyes deep with sympathy. He said something to my mother about my still being "intact," but that he had injected spermicide to make sure I didn't become pregnant.

"Thank *god*," she said, with what sounded like an almost primal sense of relief.

Neither the doctor nor my mother talked to me. They were talking over me, around me.

They couldn't even look at me.

The next day my mother kept me home from school. She said we had another appointment. We drove downtown to Buffalo's police headquarters, where we met a middle-aged policewoman in a grimy office under neon lights. With an artificial smile, partially concealed under lips covered in bright red lipstick, she settled behind a gray Royal typewriter and rolled in several pieces of paper with dark sheets of carbon to make duplicates. She announced that she needed the details—*all* the details—of what happened to me.

"A crime has occurred," she said. "You must make a statement."

She had to question me to get as much information as possible.

The policewoman went over the previous afternoon, minute by minute. Every time I said something, she listened, typed, then asked more questions.

I grew more and more tense. Speaking aloud about what happened, without euphemisms, going over the incident in all its ugliness, made it even more terrifying, filling the room with its menace. I had no power in this room, in my life, and yet now I was being ordered to describe every detail of the worst thing ever to happen to me—to a complete stranger? *Why?* I thought. *Why do I have to? Why don't I matter, right now, or ever?*

But her questions continued. They fell like hammer blows to my head, over and over.

When it came to the verge of describing the sexual act itself, I stopped talking. The room thundered with silence. My mother, pale and drawn, said nothing.

"Well?"

I said nothing.

The policewoman prompted, with false jocularity, "Come on now, we're all girls!"

She was trying to make me relax, to ease the answers out of me, but it was not done for me or for my comfort. She had a job to do, information to extract.

Her questions became more and more insistent.

My mother stayed silent.

I finally resumed talking, but as I did, I felt like I was being attacked all over again.

What I wanted, or thought, or felt, was beside the point. I had to make a statement. It made no difference if I were ready.

The details chipped away at my only protection: My belief, against overwhelming evidence to the contrary, that life would someday achieve a level of calm, and worry would be a thing of the past.

CHAPTER 26

THE SEARCH

IN ALL THE JUVENILE BIOGRAPHIES OF FAMOUS PEOPLE THAT I LOVED TO READ IN the children's section of the nearby public library, nothing so horrible had ever happened to anyone famous. Even the few books about famous women that I read, over and over—"Marie Curie, Girl Scientist," or "Maria Mitchell, Girl Astronomer"—they were never attacked and dragged into bushes.

This fact made me feel even more alone.

Why am I so different? I thought. *Why did this happen?*

Years would pass before I understood how much awful company I had, how I had joined a grim sisterhood. Sexual assaults of women and girls were as common as dirt, but in 1969, such incidents were blanketed in denial, minimized, disparaged, ignored, rarely published in newspapers, and almost never spoken of in any honest way.

"You can tell me," the policewoman coaxed. Slowly, falteringly, I spoke. I groped for words. I felt waves and waves of shame. She typed as I talked. In my narrative, I said the man took down my underwear.

The policewoman stopped.

"You mean panties," she said.

"No, I mean underwear," I replied.

The policewoman shook her head. Her mouth tightened.

"Panties," she said, firmly.

This made me even more upset. *Why aren't my words good enough? I thought. Whose statement is this? And what are panties anyway? Isn't that something pretty and lacy? Nobody ever referred to the white, cotton underwear I wore as "panties."*

"Uh, I guess so," I said, finally.

She smiled and resumed typing. When the relentless bludgeoning of her questions finally stopped, she unrolled the sheets of paper out of the typewriter and displayed them with obvious pride. There it was: my nightmare, in triplicate.

Yet, in what was supposed to be my statement, she had typed the word "panties" throughout the narrative.

The word enraged me. I felt like taking a pen and crossing the word out wherever it appeared, over and over, the pen slashing so deep it would rip the paper. I wanted to tear the pages into a thousand pieces.

But I was silent.

We left the police department and entered a gray afternoon with the bite of frost already on the wind. To escape the chill, we ducked into a restaurant for lunch. My mother said I could have anything I wanted. This almost never happened. I ordered meatloaf, mashed potatoes, and green beans. But I could barely eat half. The potatoes, normally my favorite, stuck in my throat.

The experience of that day, and the day before, washed over me like waves, crashing over and over.

We said little to one another for the rest of the meal. We didn't talk about the scene in the police station.

Later that night, my father upbraided her.

"You could have prevented the attack. You let the kids do whatever the hell they want. You don't know where they are half the time."

I could feel his anger pulsing through the walls.

He didn't say that he didn't even realize where I was when I left his office.

He didn't say that he could have taken the few minutes to drive me the five blocks home.

He didn't say, "Honey, we will get through this somehow."

My mother, defensive and grief-stricken, began to monitor my activities. She told me to walk home with all the other kids after school.

"Walk with your friends," she insisted.

I didn't point out I had no friends.

"Don't swim after school. Don't go to Dad's office."

Although we never spoke about the assault directly after that, a week after my father levied accusations against her, my mother erupted, saying angrily, "I told you not to go into that lot. I told you."

I realized that Ellen must have felt the same way about her illness and I glimpsed the awful burden she carried. We had something in common. Something was happening to both of us that was frightening—leaden, dragging us down, and yet must somehow remain unsaid lest it become even more powerful.

I knew what my role was. My responsibility was to make everyone else feel better. *Just pretend that everything is all right*, I told myself. I could make my mother feel better. I had to.

After school, I spoke with an artificial cheerfulness. I made up imaginary conversations with friends that I didn't have. I would emphasize trivial news.

"Sister Mary Vincent's cat had kittens!" I would relate with a gaiety I didn't feel. It was astonishing how few lies it took to reassure my mother. Soon, she began to lose her drawn, pinched look. My mother smiled more.

I overheard her talk about it to my sister Claudia.

"Kids are so resilient. They bounce back from bad events so much more easily than adults. She'll be fine."

Claudia, five years older than me and a senior in high school, said something noncommittal. She was the only person in my world who refused to say that everything would be all right.

As time passed, my tap dancing continued.

"See?" my actions said. "Everything is fine. The rape? That little thing? I've forgotten all about it.

"Everything is going just as well as can be expected."

When I was not putting on an act, at odd moments, I got even quieter than usual, often staring off into space. Nobody seemed to notice, except Claudia.

One night, she put her arms around me.

"I know you are upset about what happened to you," she whispered. "I know you feel humiliated. You can talk about it if you want to."

She held me for a long time.

But I didn't talk about it.

The incident was always at the back of my mind, though—background music of a horror show that never seemed to end. Some days the assault crowded out all other thoughts. I woke up with it. I dreamt about it. The man. The bushes. The smell of autumn leaves.

The fear.

Every time I came close to forgetting for a while, the police would show up unannounced at our house. There was nothing subtle about these visits. They, in fact, could not have been more ham-handed, their actions seemingly designed to inflict more humiliation. They never arrived in an unmarked car. They would park their police cruiser in front of the house and wait for me to come home from school. They never wore civilian clothes, either.

The police were usually young and earnest. They wanted to catch my assailant. They were convinced he lived somewhere in the area. But to find him, they insisted, required driving around the neighborhood with me in the back seat of their police cruiser, scanning the streets, on the next-to-zero chance that I would see my assailant. Then, presumably, they would sprint out of their cruiser and arrest him.

I thought the idea was idiotic.

Catching him was the right thing to try to do, though, I knew that. Otherwise, he could hurt another little girl.

When I got an A in English, or did a math problem correctly on the chalkboard in front of the class after the teacher randomly called on me, I felt a rare sense of triumph.

But each time I saw the police cruiser crouched outside the house, my little spark of joy was snuffed out, turning it, instantly, to dread. The day turned to dust. The assault crashed in on me. It began to smother me once again. The hard ground. The gag. The smirk.

I worried that neighbors would think I was being arrested— repeatedly. Would they think I was a juvenile delinquent, seeing me in the back seat of a cruiser over and over again?

My depression deepened. The idea that everything was fine became harder to believe in.

Keep dancing, I thought. *Or everything will fall apart.*

Otherwise, my parents would fight about what happened. My mother would be sad; not just about Ellen, but me, too. I had to convince everyone that I was OK. At least Claudia knew the truth: I was far from OK. But I couldn't talk about it, even with her.

A month later, in social studies class, the assault began to dominate my thoughts, replaying over and over on an endless loop in my mind. As I ruminated, I felt like I was drowning in despair.

The teacher's voice telescoped, becoming fainter and fainter. And the classroom faded around me. I was falling, falling, deep into darkness. It was a Pit, one just for me.

I am dying, I thought. *This is how people feel at the very end of their lives.*

It was strangely familiar.

No light came to this place. I heard no angels.

Still, in the blackness I felt a Presence all around me, holding me tight against my own despair.

It was not Jesus. I did not see the dove of the Holy Spirit. It was simply a knowing, a realization that Someone was here, right here.

And in that abyss God whispered to me.

"I am with you in this dark, dark night."

I sensed immediately that when I was attacked, when I experienced that evil, that God was the first to weep. I stayed there for a long time, and let the Presence hold me close and felt—for the first time—comfort.

Slowly, the teacher's voice returned, and I emerged from the Pit, light breaking through. I could see the classroom once again. I didn't know how long I was away. Minutes? Seconds?

But God remained—quiet, steadfast.

At night, in the silence, my sense of the Presence continued.

Lying in my bed, I felt the truth of what I was to read, years later, in Dante's *Paradiso:* "God is the love that moves the sun and the other stars."

Eventually, the police stopped waiting for me after school. The atmosphere of the house returned to our version of normal. I began to have more days in which I didn't think about what happened.

A year passed. Then, I saw him.

On that afternoon, the laundromat around the corner from my house featured hot air, dirty clothes, and my rapist.

He had the same dark hair, same five o'clock shadow. He was jumping up and down to music on a small transistor radio, arms flailing, head bouncing, singing like an imbecile.

He's nuts, I thought, instantly. *He is truly insane.*

And then he saw me, through the large, dirty pane glass windows of the laundromat.

In the same moment, by sheer force of will, I controlled my facial expression and pretended I did not see him.

Yet I did. And here, in a public place, among people bustling to businesses, I did not feel afraid.

The tables had turned. He was afraid of *me.*

His face became pale. His eyes grew wide. He stopped smiling and dancing, and turned off his radio.

I instantly understood the decision I faced. I walked to the convenience store nearest the laundromat and stepped into its alcove, pressing myself against the brick wall of the building, out of sight.

In that moment I knew that I could, and should, call the police. But then the cycle of waiting cruisers, interviews, humiliation, and dark memories would begin all over again.

It had been a year. Even if the police arrived quickly enough to find him and arrest him, would the charges stick? Would I survive months of visiting, in my mind, the images that had tormented me? Would I have to testify in front of a judge and jury, airing for everyone the worst day of my life for their questioning, their examination? Would it be my word against his? Would anyone believe me?

Calling the police was the right thing to do. It was the moral choice. If they caught him, maybe he would go to prison. Maybe he would not hurt another girl.

But the process was guaranteed to be awful.

What would I get out of it besides more depression, more suffering?

Yet my religion, my family culture, had conditioned me for years to put myself, my own needs, last.

I must think of others, I thought.

Still.

What about me?

I stayed in the alcove, still, and waited.

The man emerged from the laundromat, springing from the front door like a parasite bursting from its host. He was no longer dancing. He was utterly frantic. He looked both ways at the traffic and pealed across Elmwood Avenue, threading between honking cars. He sprinted down the street until I no longer saw him.

I let out my breath, not realizing until then that I had been holding it.

Call the police?

Hell no.

I walked back home and told no one what I had seen.

CHAPTER 27

THE CURE-ALL ELIXIR

WORRIES OF SEEING MY ASSAILANT AGAIN DISSIPATED. HIS NERVOUSNESS, HIS fear, had emboldened me. I wasn't afraid of him. I was afraid, however, of being assaulted again by some unknown man.

I envied my brothers' freedom. They never worried about walking home, even at night. Their bodies protected them. Mine would always put me at risk. I now understood that I shared a searing experience, a knowledge of my own vulnerability, that unites women everywhere. If the night was beautiful, it still held dangers. If streets seem quiet, we still are forced to remain vigilant. Women are robbed of serenity because we are targets. *I was once,* I fretted. *Would I be again?*

I rarely felt safe in the city after I was attacked.

One of the few times I felt completely out of harm's way was when one of Ellen's doctors, Mary Hawking, hired me to walk her dog. She was a brilliant physician, but I basked in her attention and her kindness. She was one medical professional who didn't shrink from becoming a friend to patient families, including ours.

When Dr. Hawking contemplated accepting a residency in the United States from her native Great Britain, she thought about the crime rate and considered what a single woman, living alone, could do to protect herself. She saw only two choices: Get a dog or buy a gun. She got a black German Shepherd puppy with huge paws that soon grew to the biggest, most ferocious-looking animal most of us had ever seen. Yet, Bran was sweet and gentle, even though he was nearly big enough for me to ride.

I inherited the dog-walking job from Ellen, when her hospitalizations became too frequent for her to continue. It was good pay at fifty cents an hour. Even better, walking Bran gave me the experience of freedom and complete safety for which I longed. Nobody would bother me with Bran trotting beside me. Even so, I experienced an increasing amount of unwanted attention from men in the form of shouted catcalls or whistles from drivers. I pretended to ignore them, but the attention was intimidating.

Without Bran, I got into the habit of looking over my shoulder regularly when I walked anywhere. That hyper-awareness saved me. Twice, over several years, men tried to grab me on the street a few blocks from my house, but both times I shoved them, hard, and got away. Another man exposed himself one night as I rounded the corner from the nearby stores; I ran into the house. The incidents were tremendously upsetting, but I told no one. Instead, I began to take karate lessons at the Jewish Center just to feel less vulnerable.

However, I soon developed my preferred method of coping with the tension of Ellen's illness and the fear that I would be attacked again.

I began to drink.

I had always helped myself to random sips of wine or beer. My parents thought nothing of it. Drinking a full glass was a ritual reserved for adulthood. My brother Seamus ended that mystery one night in the city. We were both sitting on the porch, watching rain come down in sheets. He, at twenty, decided that I, at thirteen, was old enough to learn how to handle alcohol. My heart leapt at this compliment. Flattery that he, the oldest, trusted me to drink far exceeded my curiosity about the beer itself. It was an honor. He opened a full, cold bottle of Genesee Cream Ale and handed it to me.

It was magic.

Every tension, every fear in my life washed away in moments. Haunting memories from my assault melted. Dad's raging at home became a mere curiosity and lost its edge. My loneliness at school seemed trivial next to this floating feeling of happiness.

I giggled uncontrollably.

With that brown bottle came the confidence that everything would work out. Ellen would live. I would make friends. People would stop teasing me at school. I would be safe. Dad would stop yelling. The rain stopped and I began to run back and forth across the street, jumping in puddles and splashing, just to express the newfound energy, the uncontrolled joy, I felt. Seamus laughed as he watched me, putting his feet up on the porch balustrade and downing his own beer.

The next morning, the effect of the alcohol had worn off. But it didn't matter. I had the answer to all my troubles.

I couldn't wait to drink again. I began to drink with regularity, a few times a month at first, then more often. As long as I acted like it didn't affect me, it was met with unspoken approval. "Holding your liquor" was a prized attribute in our house. Pretend you were drinking water, and nobody would think twice about your habits. Alcohol was such an ingrained part of family life that it seemed natural to start years before the legal drinking age. After all, every-one knew that the best way to learn how to drink without ill effect was to start early, at home, so you could learn how to "handle it" in a safe environment. Experimenting with alcohol was considered a natural part of growing up. My parents shrugged at teen alcohol use, and so did other adults in our world. They were clueless about the impact of their beliefs around alcohol use and their own exam-ples. Their cherished convictions about booze were myths.

One of the most effective ways to develop alcoholism in adult-hood is to start drinking early in the teenage years, research shows, when the brain is undergoing rapid growth. Early alcohol use increases potential for alcohol problems later on. My own father began drinking when he was twelve.

My brother did me no favors in handing me that first bottle of beer, but another adult might have done the same soon enough. With no counseling available to help me manage my own daily experience of fear, sadness, and rage, alcohol became a warm blan-ket of solace. It was the only thing that helped me escape, even for a little while, the ever-present worry about Ellen's deteriorating health.

Her dialysis twice a week helped her survive, but her skimpy diet continued. She continued to be hospitalized without warning, off and on. One day her blood pressure would spike, and doctors would admit her. Or tests wouldn't be quite right, and she would go into the hospital for another week. I never understood what sparked these medical episodes. Some were more harrowing than others. During one traumatic event that Ellen related to me after-ward, she even had a near-death experience.

While she was in the hospital, she lost consciousness in mid-sentence and abruptly felt herself leaving her body. She told me later she hovered near the ceiling, suddenly feeling no discomfort. She watched what happened next with a detached interest. Claudia and Mom had been with her, talking. When she passed out, the machine to which she was attached began to emit loud beeps. Suddenly, the room was filled with people in white coats who frantically began to work on Ellen. Still near the ceiling, she watched as Mom became pale and Claudia's eyes widened. Then, like getting sucked into a vacuum cleaner, Ellen entered her body again and opened her eyes.

"What was it like?" I said.

"Cool. Peaceful. It felt good," she replied. "But I didn't like seeing Mom so upset."

Ellen's hospitalizations occurred so often that some weeks, the only time I could be with her was when she was at the dialysis clinic. Each time I saw her, she looked a little more shrunken, her matchstick arms bruised by the endless needles. On my visits, I brought cards so we could play rummy.

Her new plastic eye was brown, matching her good eye. She often joked about it. At night, she would take it out, clean it and put it on a table beside her bed, like a pair of dentures. I became accustomed to the sight of her empty, eyeless socket.

The sight would have scared the bullies at school, but Ellen was mostly getting tutored intermittently at home or in the hospital. Even so, she wasn't above playing practical jokes with her plastic orb.

That became apparent during a family party in South Buffalo. Ian Sullivan, a distant cousin by marriage and failed lawyer, was also in attendance. He graduated from a well-known law school but never reached his expected level of professional success. He married the prettiest girl in his neighborhood and the marriage didn't last three years. He ran for the elected position of judge and came in seventh out of seven candidates. With every failure, he drank more heavily. With every drink, he became more overbearing.

At the gathering, Ian became more boorish as the night wore on. He finished one whiskey and water and, spying Ellen, thrusted his empty glass at her.

"Get me another drink," he ordered. He didn't say please. But he did make the mistake of glancing away.

In a flash, Ellen popped out her plastic eye and dropped it, with a hollow sound, into his waiting glass.

It circled the tumbler briefly and then nestled, contented as a fake eye could be, among the whiskey-soaked ice cubes.

Ian paused for a moment. Then, feeling the sudden weight in his glass, he looked down to see Ellen's brown eyeball gazing blankly up at him amid the shards of ice.

"Oops. I wondered where I left that," Ellen said. She scooped the eye back up and popped it in her eye socket in one, smooth motion. "The alcohol will probably kill the germs, don't you think?" she asked Ian, looking innocent.

Ian's face turned green. He placed the glass on the nearest table, found a seat, and neither drank nor talked to anyone else for the rest of the gathering.

We laughed all the way home.

As she got sicker, though, her humor failed her. During one trying time, when she was fourteen, she had been in the hospital for two weeks. The stay was longer than usual. Her physical health was too fragile for her to return home, even though we only lived three blocks away. Every time she was close to being discharged, a medical crisis would occur. Then she had to stay longer.

None of Ellen's elaborate distractions worked for her anymore. She became listless and depressed. Summer was near and she wanted to go to the cottage. Instead, she was in a glass and brick edifice, on the fifth floor once again, poked and prodded and no closer to getting well than she had been for three years.

The more discouraged Ellen became, the worse her lab reports turned out.

She got sicker and sicker, and slipped further away from her goal of coming home.

My parents became frantic.

At home, Mom openly worried that we were losing her.

Dad didn't know what to do. Morose, he began to show up in her hospital room at 2 a.m. He would sit in her room, in the dark, sighing heavily and filling the room with the smell of secondhand alcohol.

"Ellie? Are you awake? I'll just sit here for awhile, honey," he would whisper.

"OK, Dad," Ellen would reply. She said she never minded his middle-of-the-night visits, but the hospital staff was outraged, and finally told him to confine his visits to daylight so Ellen could get more sleep.

Her deterioration continued, and it seemed as though nobody had an answer.

But Seamus did. To him, the problem was obvious.

"She's depressed," he said. "She can't get better while she feels this way. She needs something to live for."

One early evening, he called the nurses on the fifth floor, all of whom we knew by then, and asked them to bring Ellen down to the hospital lobby at 8:30 p.m. That was when their supervisor, who would have forbidden the mission, ate dinner. She would be conveniently out of the way. After Seamus explained his plan, the nurses agreed immediately.

He asked me to come with him.

We walked into the silent, empty lobby, so different from its usual daytime bustle, and we waited. Finally, the elevator doors opened. Ellen looked shrunken in a wheelchair, wearing jeans and a tee shirt. She was totally confused.

"What's going on?" she said, gesturing to the smiling nurses. "They won't tell me anything."

Seamus held a laundry basket he had brought from home, covered in a blanket.

"Here," he said. "Take a look at this."

Mystified, but intrigued, Ellen pulled off the blanket.

A Belgian shepherd puppy squirmed out, curly tail wagging furiously, black and brown and full of energy. She put her paws on Ellen's thin chest and licked her chin.

Ellen's face lit up.

"A dog! You got me a dog!" she said, over and over. The puppy wriggled as she pet her. The nurses had tears in their eyes.

"She's yours, but you have to get better," Seamus said. "You have to get out of the hospital to take care of her. She doesn't even have a name! You have to think of one. She doesn't know how to do anything. You have to train her. Can you do that?"

"Yes, oh, yes," Ellen said, over and over, laughing and hugging the puppy, who instantly decided, as dogs do, that being with Ellen would be her mission in life. In that moment, Ellen was happier than she had been in years. She named the dog Mickey.

To the medical staff's amazement, the numbers on Ellen's lab reports, which had been deteriorating for days, suddenly made dramatic U-turns. Ellen's fragile health stabilized. The hospital released her within days.

She came home to a reunion with her beloved Mickey. For a while, there seemed no limits to the joy and improving health that a dog could give.

But Ellen's doctors knew better. They knew they were running out of time. They began to discuss the possibility of performing a then-rare operation on Ellen: a kidney transplant.

CHAPTER 28

WHEN TRANSPLANTS
WERE MIRACLES

ORGAN TRANSPLANTS WERE STILL RARE IN THE LATE 1960S. THE ORGAN DONOR network was word of mouth. There was no nationwide, organized effort to match donors and patients in desperate need.

An obstacle course of legal hurdles and bureaucracy often prevented the use of cadaver organs in transplants. Upon death, a body was the legal property of next of kin. Relatives could and often did ignore the wishes of a deceased person to be an organ donor. There were legal problems transporting organs across state boundaries, even when the borders were nearby. The Uniform Anatomical Gift Act, a law drafted in 1968 and adopted by most states within three years, helped hammer out legal procedures regarding organ donations among competing jurisdictions.

Yet, red tape was not the only problem. The moment a person dies, organs begin to deteriorate, but there was then no uniform method of establishing brain death. No wonder that doctors preferred to perform a transplant between a living relative and a lucky recipient. After all, humans are born with two kidneys, but need only one.

In Ellen's case, doctors could see the need for a transplant coming for many months. Three years into her disease, Ellen's deteriorating kidneys began to wreak even more havoc. She learned to always carry a package of tissues to stem the flow of sudden nosebleeds. She would get short of breath. Right before she turned fourteen, doctors finally removed the nearly dead kidneys in an operation that even my stoic sister said was excruciating once the anesthesia had worn off. Once the kidneys were gone, there was no turning back. A transplant was her only hope of surviving into adulthood.

The first major experiments with transplants took place early in the twentieth century. The brilliant French surgeon, Alexis Carrel, won a Nobel Prize as early as 1912 for improving surgical techniques, but he also transplanted kidneys between dogs. He figured out that rejection was an immune system response. But there was no real progress toward transplanting organs until the 1940s.

That occurred when a young physician named Joseph Murray became involved with treating servicemen who had catastrophic burns and applied what he learned about skin graft rejection to experiments with organ transplants. Murray performed the first successful kidney transplant between identical twins in December, 1954.

Transplants between twins were simple, though, compared to the daunting hurdles that the same operation posed between non-identical humans. To suppress the immune system for recipients not lucky enough to have a twin donor, Murray and his colleagues relied on total-body irradiation to give the transplanted kidney a chance to function without the body rejecting the foreign organ—a risky, dangerous technique prone to failure. Only by late 1963 did the nascent transplant field discover that a combination of prednisone, a steroid, and Imuran could fight rejection. With that breakthrough, two dozen medical centers began doing transplants the following year.

Yet, one of the biggest obstacles to treatment and the operation itself had nothing to do with medical care, but the ongoing bane of the American health care system: the need for money. Treating chronic kidney disease, keeping patients alive on dialysis, preparing for and conducting transplants, and the necessary aftercare were all prohibitively expensive.

Until this point, insurance covered the cost of Ellen's care through our father's job. But our luck was about to run out.

As if anticipating Ellen's need for an expensive transplant, the health insurance company sent our parents a letter about Ellen's medical bills. In legal jargon, the letter explained that Ellen's medical coverage was about to come to a screeching halt. At the moment of Ellen's greatest need, the company began the process of removing her from its rolls.

All the hospital expenses, the lab tests, the cost of twice-weekly dialysis, the frequent hospital stays, fees from specialists, the overwhelming blizzard of bills that Ellen's devastating illness created would suddenly no longer be the responsibility of insurance. The costs of her kidney disease had exceeded the lifetime cap of $1 million in medical bills that our insurance was legally obligated to pay for any one individual, the letter explained. Our parents would now be responsible for paying the cost of her care.

The prospect was dizzying. There was no end to the expenses of Ellen's illness. The only mystery is that it had taken several years of crises and hospital stays to add up to $1 million. The kidney transplant alone—if it ever took place—would cost tens of thousands of dollars.

My father wrote letters appealing the decision, to no avail. My mother was, in her own words, "a wreck." Any fights that my parents had over money paled next to the hammer that was about to smash every aspect of our lives. Saving Ellen was a family imperative, our shared focus. But now the money necessary to accomplish that would crush all of us. Everyone would need to get jobs, my mother told us. She worried that we would lose the house, like her parents did during the Great Depression. And there was no Aunt Lil to save us.

To our surprise, there existed an entity with bigger pockets poised to intervene. Once my mother told Ellen's doctors of the soul-crushing letter from the insurance company—hoping to negotiate lower fees—they smiled and told her not to worry. Mystified, my mother asked why. That's when she learned about a New York State program everyone referred to simply as "state aid."

In 1969, New York, the object of derision, resentment, and even contempt in many corners of the country for its high taxes, had taxpayer-funded programs to help people like us. Doctors told my parents that New York had provisions to assist middle-class people whose health insurance proved inadequate for the cost of a catastrophic illness. It took a few phone calls, and some paperwork signed by the hospital's chief physician to enroll Ellen in the program.

It was a miracle imbedded in the remnants and compassion of New Deal politics that cared about people, not just business. Organized, corporate resentment and companies' elected mouthpieces had not yet managed to erode this approach. The payment of Ellen's medical bills moved from insurance coverage to the public purse. The transition was seamless.

After state officials processed the paperwork, my family never saw a bill for Ellen's ever-more-expensive medical care. Ellen could be saved, not because of her personality, her potential, her ethnicity, skin color, religion, political connections, whom our parents knew or what they thought, but through the accident of state residency—the random blessing of geography. My parents never lost the house. No child labor was necessary to pay the endless bills. A transplant, if it were even possible, would surely be a risk on many levels, but it would not be a financial roll of the dice. New York state taxpayers would pay for Ellen's care.

Big government was our hero.

In 1970, around four hundred kidney transplants in the United States took place between living donors and relatives. Twice as many operations used cadaver kidneys, even though they had a higher failure rate than organs from living relatives. The operation had become somewhat more common, but the field was still in its infancy. Ellen's doctors had a lot to consider.

In 1970, the one-year survival rate of transplanted kidneys from a parent to a child was above 70 percent, in part because children share molecules called antigens with both parents. If Ellen got a kidney from one of our parents, her immune system would see similar antigens in the donor organ and treat them as friends rather than hostile invaders, making rejection of the new kidney less likely.

But Ellen's odds would plunge if a cadaver kidney was her only hope. The one-year survival rate of donated, cadaver kidneys was around 40 percent after two years in 1970, with the still-limited understanding of all the variables necessary to successfully match a patient with an unrelated donor. Seventy percent of patients receiving a cadaver kidney needed dialysis after transplantation.

Even finding a cadaver kidney was difficult. Matching a donor with a recipient required calling individual hospitals, and at the time there were about four hundred in New York State. The state Health Department announced a plan to use a central computer in Albany connected to a teletype in each hospital to match donor kidneys with patients, but the complex system would take many months to implement.

We didn't dwell on a cadaver kidney as an option. We were hopeful that one of us could give a kidney to Ellen. The size of our family, with seven potential donors, made us optimistic. That meant there were fourteen kidneys for a potential organ harvest. I thought of my family as a kind of fruit tree, with kidneys hanging from every branch.

Surely one of them could work out.

In the spring of 1970, with great fanfare and a welcome day away from school, Ellen's doctors arranged for all of us to take blood tests to see who would be the best donor.

The tests confirmed what my mother had already told the medical team: Mom's blood type was O positive; Dad's was A positive. The rest of our blood types occurred in a distinct pattern, like rungs of a ladder, from oldest to youngest. Seamus, Claudia and Ellen all had O blood type; the rest of us had A.

Only those with an O blood type could be potential donors.

My chance at saving Ellen melted away. But I wasn't the only one. Soon after, my mother said that none of the girls could donate. We were not beyond "childbearing age." She told us that doctors feared that having only one kidney might interfere with our ability to someday bear children. This was untrue, I found out later.

Mom had more excuses when it came to my brother Seamus's ability to donate. Unlike me, he had O positive blood—the same as Ellen's. Also, he was twenty and in excellent physical health. But

Mom argued that the operation would interfere with his athletics, even though rowing was not a contact sport.

In this game of medical musical chairs, my mother made sure there was only one possible source of a life-giving kidney left standing: herself. She marshaled the facts and arguments to make certain that she would be the one to take the risk. In the decades since, significantly more women than men have also become living transplant donors. Mom's thinking was no different than tens of thousands of mothers who followed in her footsteps.

Yet, this was so early in the evolution of kidney transplants that every discussion felt like we were preparing to walk on the moon.

With a compatible blood type and as Ellen's parent, Mom had advantages as a donor. But she offered disadvantages, too. My mother would be forty-eight by the time the transplant took place in the fall. She had smoked for most of her adult life. She had a lung and a half and a heart murmur. Behind closed doors, doctors debated the feasibility of using Mom's kidney. Ellen's situation, never stable, continued to decline. Her need for a transplant was immediate.

Given my mother's devotion to prayer, it's unfortunate that none of us knew about the saints Cosmas and Damian, physician twins who traveled throughout the Roman world in the late third century after the death of Christ and healed the sick through their medical skills.

According to legend, the twins used a leg from a deceased gladiator to replace the diseased leg of a dying patient. Thus, they accomplished all those centuries ago what is even today beyond medical science, earning their status as the patron saints of the medical transplantation field.

Surely, had we known, we would have prayed ceaselessly to help speed the transplant and ensure its success. But even without the twins' example, we had no doubts that Ellen's salvation was at hand.

Ellen and I didn't think about the odds against her. We paid no heed to the likelihood that, even if the transplant went off without a hitch, Ellen's body might reject the organ. We believed in happy endings: All of Ellen's suffering, her patience, her stoicism, would be rewarded in the end. The operation meant that everything would be all right. Life would go back to the peaceful days of 1966. All would be as it once was.

CHAPTER 29

PINING TO SAIL

BETWEEN THE UNCERTAIN PRESENT AND THE HOPE OF A TRANSPLANT THAT COULD be Ellen's salvation in the fall, there was summer and the quiet island that awaited us.

While the rest of us looked forward to a much-needed rest, Ellen struggled. For her, sheer determination, and short rests, were the only way she found the energy to climb the steep stairs leading from the docks up to the cottages, insisting all the way that she didn't need any help.

But once at the top of the stairs, there was only a short walk to the cottage. If we arrived in the afternoon and she had the energy, Ellen and I would then walk to one of the nearby stony beaches where we would collect driftwood for one of our evening bonfires.

Ellen and I organized little in our lives, but when it came to planning an evening on the beach, we became bonfire engineers. We tried to set up the wood so the fire would start with just one match. We would carefully stack the kindling like Lincoln logs, twigs and dried grass at the bottom, with ever-larger pieces of twisted timber on top. We would roll logs that were scattered on the beach and set them up around where our fire would blaze at night. The logs, bleached white, were comfortable to rest against, their surfaces sanded smooth by weather and water.

After the sky began to darken, past 9 p.m. on summer nights, Ellen and I and anyone else who wanted to join us would trek to the beach, pulling a wagon with provisions: corn and potatoes to cook in glowing coals; marshmallows for roasting; towels, in case we wanted to go for a night swim; blankets to lay down over the ever-present rocks; jars of Kool-Aid; silverware; and flashlights so we could safely descend to the rocky shore.

The beach was always quiet. Most of the island population preferred to relax at night in their cottages watching TV rather than linger on a deserted beach. No sound intruded on our little oasis, except the restless waves and soon, fire crackling from the wood we had so carefully arranged hours before.

Most nights, though, it was just Ellen and me. We would dip ears of corn in the waters of the lake and roll them on a bed of embers to steam in their own leaves, later savoring their sweet, smoky flavor. We would gaze across the water and talk about the future, until the years to come seemed as bright as the moon shining on the breakers. The fire would slowly die, our conversation would quiet, and we would finally douse the blaze, the fire hissing in protest as it reluctantly dimmed and disappeared.

With the beach enveloped in darkness once again, and no lights to dim the stars, the whole universe soared above, silent and majestic. There was no telling what drama the night sky would unfurl. In August, the shooting stars of the Perseids would appear, our own fireworks, meteors silently streaking to Earth, some falling in

clusters or individually, like jewels dropping from a broken neck-
lace one by one. On one memorable evening, when we braved the
April chill to stay in the cottage overnight, the northern lights
descended with flickering, green curtains over Lake Ontario, waving silently as if blown by winds sweeping across the solar system.
The colors above reflected on the waters below, and the night, brit-
tle with cold, blazed with light.

The warmth of summer, though, made it easy to star gaze for
endless hours. The sky during some summer nights was far too
beautiful to waste on sleep. When the stars were particularly daz-
zling, I would launch a rowboat into the quiet harbor. Lying across
the middle seat as the boat drifted slowly in the current, gazing
upwards, I would listen to the occasional quacking of ducks nestled
in the reeds, the lapping of water and the wind until the wee hours
of the morning. Other aspects of my life routinely made me feel
insignificant, but never the night sky soaring above. The stars I
gazed upon had been shining for millennia. They felt like friendly
messengers, reminding me that whatever troubles I had were temporary, and that just as every star had its place, so did every life
have a role in the universe.

When I became too tired to gaze upward, I would tie up the
boat, slip onto the sunporch, and curl up on the fainting couch.
Sleeping on the sunporch, with its many tall, screened, but shade-
less windows, may have conditioned me to become an early riser.
Bird song after dawn was my alarm clock.

Later in the morning, I would often see a small fleet of sail-
boats gather across the harbor. The toy-like vessels were red,
green, and blue, and danced across the sun-dappled water. Kids
my age piloting the vessels zig-zagged in the late morning breeze
that would kick up a modest chop in the protected harbor. The

boats belonged to a marina that offered sailing classes for young people, which I pined to join. I watched with envy as the children learned how to handle lines, ducking under the swinging booms and yelling obscure commands like "Prepare to come about!" as the boats skimmed over the water.

I began to ask my parents if I, too, could learn to sail. My mother stalled and deflected, giving time-honored parental responses like, "We'll see," or "Maybe later," answers designed to avoid direct conflict but snuff out questions. I knew that there was almost no chance of getting permission. It was nothing personal, just a fact of life about living in a large family. We were expected to share everything—clothes, toys, and when possible, experiences. Doing anything else would threaten the family's fragile equilibrium. If I had the opportunity to learn sailing, then any one of my brothers or sisters should have a chance at the same thing. A $10 lesson for one could soon become $20 or $30.

Since all the money from Aunt Lil had petered out, there was little chance, I knew, that I would join the kids across the harbor on their dancing boats. And lessons were a slippery slope. The experience of learning to sail would lead to the next step—pestering my parents to buy a sailboat, an unthinkable request.

I tried anyway. I asked my father to pay for lessons, or at least, to teach me to sail. He had spent his youth in the Sea Scouts, sailing on Lake Erie. He would regale us with stories of sailing swiftly to beat the summer storms on that most shallow of the Great Lakes, where waves would loom large in minutes with the right wind.

"You could teach me," I wheedled. "Who needs lessons? You and I could do this together."

Dad's response fit his usual pattern. He instantly agreed.

"Yes, but not now."

"Yes, maybe later."

"Yes, of course, what father would turn down such a chance to be with his daughter?"

"We will sail to Canada!" he would say, smiling and opening a beer. "We will pick a nice day, when the waves aren't too high. With the right wind, it would only take five hours!"

"When?" I would ask, thrilled at the prospect.

"Soon!" Dad would reply, taking a long swig of his beer.

He was the prince of promises, and our relationship was littered with their bones. He would promise trips, toys, and time together. But his pledges were the illusion of action. They came with a catch. When he promised something, we were supposed to leave him alone. He would get around to fulfilling his pledges in his own good time. Yet that time never came. This fact was something that no polite child could readily point out without risking the appearance of insolence. I learned not to mention such unpleasant details, because I knew that his promises were to be considered almost as good as actions. The promises were signals to have faith in him, and just as important, to drop the subject. They were, in their own way, like the ending of the Mass, when the priest turned to the congregation and said, "Go in peace," the signal for the faithful to dutifully shuffle out the door.

But I wouldn't drop the idea of a sailboat.

So finally, one day, when he'd had enough of my incessant begging, Dad called the cottage before he drove in from the city. He said he had a boat for me. He had seen it at a department store, and he would bring it up to the cottage that very afternoon. He sounded pleased, and said he didn't want to disappoint me.

My heart raced. I pictured a boat—my own boat—that I could take out whenever I wanted to. Dad didn't say it was a sailboat, but he knew how much I wanted one. I hoped that it had a place for oars. Maybe I could take the mast down and use it for fishing, too.

That day, my father lugged his purchase up the stairs from the dock to the cottage and showed it to me proudly.

"See?" he said. "I told you I would get you a boat."

The vessel was flimsy, red, and boat-shaped, about five feet long, and made of very thin plastic. It had no oarlocks for oars, no paddles, no fitting for a mast, and no seats. It was, in fact, not a boat. It was a wading pool for toddlers pretending to be sailors.

"How will we sail it?" I said, looking at it dubiously. I wasn't sure it would hold me, let alone Dad.

"We'll figure it out," Dad promised. "You'll see."

In the days that followed, the boat-shaped wading pool sat on the lawn outside the cottage collecting rainwater.

My moods swung between disappointment and hope. *It wouldn't work*, I thought. It wasn't a boat. But on second thought, I considered I was wrong.

Dad, I reasoned, was a sailor. He knew what he was doing. If he said it was a boat, maybe he could see something in it that I couldn't. Maybe it was just me. Maybe I didn't have the vision that he did. I decided to test that theory by dragging the unwieldy, plastic vessel down to a beach at the end of the Island, near the long pier that marked the entrance to the harbor. I was determined to put it in the water. The boat wasn't anything close to what I had envisioned, but I was going to try to launch it anyway.

I managed to crawl in the craft and push it off the beach. My weight made it sink to within a few inches of the waterline, but it was a quiet day on the lake, and the water was still. We had an extra paddle, but the vessel was so flimsy that if I paddled too hard on one side, the boat would spin like a top. I was disappointed. But maybe I just needed more faith.

I had made it just beyond the long pier at the end of the Island and about a hundred yards away from its rusted, metal side when a motorboat came roaring by. Its wake would have been nothing for a real vessel, like the heavy wooden rowboats that we used to rent, but the plastic thing I was floating on was not meant to hold anyone larger than a toddler—on land. The fragile craft was abeam to the wake when it reached me. It might as well have been a tidal wave. The first wave gushed over one side and swamped the flimsy craft, sinking it.

I wore no life jacket, and was easily a quarter mile off shore. My parents had never splurged for formal swimming lessons. My father swam with grace, speed, and inexhaustible energy. He could swim for a mile or more without stopping. In contrast, swimming for more than two or three minutes made me breathless. I began to doggy-paddle. The water was about fifteen to twenty feet deep, easily deep enough for me to drown.

The Island looked a thousand miles away. The pier had no handholds or ladders on the sides. Its surface was ten feet above the water. I had no choice but to swim for the shore.

I was petrified, but I remembered Dad saying that if I ever encountered trouble on the water, not to panic, but to alternate floating and swimming. I knew how to float. I needed to swim toward shore, but I knew I wouldn't have the energy to get to the beach without resting, too, so I alternated my movements. Paddle, kick, float, paddle, kick, float. I tried the long strokes I had seen Dad do so often and with such ease, but they just made me tired. Paddle, kick, float, paddle, kick, float. The shore came closer by inches. Finally, I staggered onto the beach, coughing up lake water.

I rested there for a long time before my heart slowed. One thought stood out: What Dad brought home was not a boat.

It was just another broken promise.

CHAPTER 30

THE HOPE OF BUTTERFLIES

SOON, MY FAMILY GOT THE MESSAGE WE HAD ALL PRAYED FOR: DOCTORS HAD finally consented to allow our mother to donate a kidney to Ellen. She would be among the first few minors to get the life-saving operation in the Buffalo area.

She wouldn't be the first; a popular boy named Ricky, who was often at Children's Hospital along with Ellen, had gotten a kidney from his dad in the hospital's first kidney transplant. Ricky had gotten a new life. Soon Ellen would, too.

In what seemed a good omen, at the end of summer, millions of welcome visitors descended on the island.

Mornings were just gaining an autumn chill that signaled the beginning of fall. The leaves gained that dusty green look, no longer vibrant, that signaled the change soon to come in late September and early October.

But one day, without warning, the trees all turned orange on their own, without the help of the dimming sunlight that caused leaves to change color. Instead, Monarch butterflies began to flock to the Island, first in pairs, then scores, hundreds, and finally hundreds of thousands; small, benevolent orange clouds flew over our dot of land on Lake Ontario, then settled as one, as if telling one another, "This looks like a nice place to rest." The butterflies covered every branch of every tree, slowly fanning their gloriously beautiful wings. They reposed on the Adirondack chairs that overlooked the harbor. They gave the Island the appearance of autumn overnight—a rare and awe-inspiring sight.

The butterflies had somehow gotten blown off course in their annual north-south migration, settling on the Island for several days before moving on in their journey to Mexico. They had never come before, and we would never experience it again.

The Island transformed overnight. No photograph could truly convey the beauty of being surrounded with trees heavy, and yet somehow light, with the gentle presence of so many glorious and delicate creatures covering every spare inch.

Ellen and I reveled in the transformation.

"They should be called flutter-bys," she marveled.

If we needed a sign that everything would work out, here it was. The unusual visit was a blessing, I thought. The butterflies foretold that the transplant to come would restore all that was good in our lives that her illness had taken away. It was easy to feel like miracles were possible because, without warning, we were living in one. The sight inspired not only awe, but optimism. So as we packed to return to the city, the hope of the butterflies filled our hearts.

CHAPTER 31

THE TRANSPLANT

LONG BEFORE THE DAY OF THE TRANSPLANT I DECIDED THAT, WHEN THE TIME came, I would skip school. Eighth grade had just begun. I didn't want to risk asking my parents for permission to stay home. There was no way I could concentrate on math or social studies when a life-changing operation involving my mother and my sister was taking place just a few blocks away.

Besides, school was just as miserable as it had ever been, only worse. The bullies that eighth-grade year grew bolder as I continued to ignore their torment.

Instead, that September morning, I got up as usual, ate breakfast, dressed in my green plaid uniform, and said goodbye to my father, who was preparing to go to work. I walked out of the front door, books under my arm. Then I turned left instead of right, walked around the house, quietly opened the side door, crept up the back stairs to the attic, and waited. Soon, my father left for work, and I walked the three blocks to Children's Hospital.

I hung around the lobby, knowing that somewhere above my mother was giving up a kidney to save the life of her daughter.

Nothing about the operation was simple.

Laparoscopic kidney removal, with its small incisions, was decades in the future. Mom had told me that surgeons would have to cut through her back muscles to take out her right kidney. The operation was highly invasive, and she would take a long time to recover.

Once Mom's kidney was removed, it would be Ellen's turn. Her doctors wouldn't put the organ back where they had removed her kidneys the previous year. Instead, they would turn over the kidney and place it in front, above Ellen's groin, with easier access to the bladder. After attaching veins and arteries, a tube called the ureter in Mom's kidney would then be attached to Ellen's bladder. Once the procedure was finished, doctors would remove the clamps and Ellen's blood would course through the kidney, now Ellen's own. We hoped, in time, it would start to produce urine.

My thoughts raced and I couldn't sit still. I lingered in the lobby for about five hours, sometimes pacing, sometimes trying to read a book but mostly re-reading the same page over and over again. Finally, a medical resident came out of the elevator whom I recognized. I always noticed her; she was the only female doctor I had ever met besides Mary Hawking.

"Maura! What are you doing here? Are you worried about your sister and your mom?"

When I nodded, without a word, she smiled.

"Relax. Your mom's kidney began to work for Ellen a half hour after the operation!"

I sank in my chair, weak with relief. It was happening. The intervention we had prayed for, hoped for against all odds, was here.

I walked home, tears filling my eyes. Irrepressible Ellen, undaunted after years of illness, and my mother, the relentless optimist, had pulled off a miracle.

Yet, unbeknownst to us, things at the hospital weren't going well. Ellen was fine. My mother wasn't.

CHAPTER 32

STRETCH MARKS

MOM'S DONATED KIDNEY, NESTLED IN ELLEN'S BODY, HAD AN IMMEDIATE, positive impact on her health. Through the glass of the intensive care unit that separated us, we saw that Ellen's gray pallor had disappeared and she now had the rosy hue of years before. We were elated.

While Ellen's new arrival couldn't have been more content, Mom's remaining kidney shut down immediately after the transplant, as if in protest that its lifelong companion had departed. For days, while she recovered from the painful procedure, she produced no urine at all. Her uremia levels rose, and the doctors grew increasingly concerned. Then, just as she seemed destined to take Ellen's empty chair in the dialysis clinic, Mom's remaining kidney chugged to life again, like an old car engine finally turning over in the cold.

The day Ellen and Mom came home felt like all of our birthdays combined into one. There were balloons and laughter; we stacked the many get well cards and notes into piles for both of them to open. For a change, we kids had cleaned up the house without complaint, mopping floors, putting away clutter, and doing the dishes, so Mom wouldn't feel like she had to do anything right away.

Our house was the worst possible place for anyone to recover from surgery. The stairs were steep, numerous, and the only bathroom was on the second floor, so we brought food up to her in trays while she healed.

She was thrilled that the kidney she donated was working and was proud of her gift to Ellen. Dr. Hardy's voodoo-like pronouncement years before stopped haunting me. Ellen would indeed live to see eighteen, and beyond. She would survive to adulthood. She could someday pursue a satisfying career, marry perhaps, and have a life.

All of us were swept up in the joy of Ellen's sudden health, but there were no parties, no sudden influx of celebrating relatives and neighbors, because she had to avoid infections. Ellen still didn't have a normal, teenage life. She couldn't attend school or see friends. Tutoring at home began again. Throwing a football with Seamus and Tim would have to wait.

But now she could eat! We could have family dinners and, except for maintaining a low-salt diet, Ellen could have almost-normal meals. No longer did any of us have to feel guilty as Ellen sliced a tiny square of steak into ten little bites. She didn't have to drink by the teaspoon. Yes, she had to keep track of her liquids, and how much urine she expelled, but her days of chronic thirst and dry, cracked lips were done.

I had so convinced myself that everything would go back to normal, where Ellen and I would go back to something resembling our old roles before her disease had upended our lives years before.

She would go back to being my older sister—mischievous, energetic, charismatic, and loud. I would become her follower again, my familiar and safe role. I could stop feeling guilty about my good health, my ability to eat and drink, the burgeoning energy I felt as I rose early every morning. She would return to robust health, a normal appetite, school, and her accustomed popularity.

Yet, like the wicked fairy who shows up, uninvited, at a christening to curse the joy of new life, a shadow fell over Ellen's new beginning. It became apparent soon after the transplant.

Ellen took an immunosuppressive drug and a steroid to fight inflammation. She would be on these drugs for years to come. The initial prescribed dose of steroids Ellen took was massive. More than 48 mg every day is considered a high dose. After the transplant, Ellen's daily dose was 200 mg. Steroids are crude tools by today's standards, but back in the fall of 1970 they were the only drugs to help fight rejection. Miraculous alternatives now taken for granted were years away.

High doses were required, and they carried risks. But there was no other choice. If Ellen rejected the kidney, it would be devastating to everyone.

The trials of the disease, and then the huge doses of steroids, stunted her growth. Although Mom once thought she was destined to be the tallest of her four girls, Ellen would instead be the smallest. She would never grow taller than five feet, one inch.

She soon developed steroid-induced diabetes and needed daily injections of insulin, which I became proficient at giving. I felt important as I swabbed her skin with alcohol and, after a quick jab, injected the life-sustaining medication. Another side effect was increased appetite. She soon gained weight and acquired the moon-like face so typical of those who are on steroids. But it was far better, we thought, than the hollow cheeks and gaunt face of hunger.

The worst side effect, though, blindsided all of us. Stretch marks appeared as soon as Ellen gained weight.

Ellen had been about seventy-six pounds when she had the transplant at fourteen. Her stick-like arms and skeletal legs were an ever-present, painful reminder of the disease and the near-starvation necessary to fight it. The sight and knowledge of her suffering so disturbed my mother that she destroyed every single photograph taken of Ellen while she was ill, save one that she had overlooked. It was as if Mom thought that ripping up photos of Ellen's life would erase the reality of the clinics, the pills, the thirst, the hunger, the dozens of hospitalizations, the emergencies, the fear, the dread, and the longing that dominated those four years. Depriving Ellen of seeing years later what she had gone through in some act of denial was ridiculous, of course.

But as Ellen gained weight, stretch marks soon snaked on Ellen's fair skin. They appeared like long, red claw marks, growing wider and longer with every passing day. The doctors called them *striae*, and seemed unfazed at their appearance. Nobody had warned us, least of all Ellen, and these angry-looking stripes were nothing close to the thin, white stretch marks some might fuss over during normal weight gain or after pregnancy.

Many were an inch wide, dark red in color, and impossible to miss or cover up with anything but clothing. They appeared everywhere on Ellen's fair skin: on the back of her legs, on the creases of her arms, on her burgeoning stomach, growing with the fat distribution from prednisone, and under her breasts. Her body, once painfully thin, now not only filled out quickly, but became unrecognizable, with long, disfiguring ribbons crisscrossing any place where a crease might form. They made the inside of her arms and backs of her legs look like she had been in some awful car accident. Soon, even on warm days, Ellen wore shirts with long sleeves and long pants.

For a girl who was just fourteen and struggling to develop a good body image after years of medical crises and an eye removal, the stretch marks must have been horrifying. For Ellen, it was like awakening after a nightmare, only to find that the bad dream was writhing and transforming itself into a new, bewildering form.

In the early days of transplants, hospitals almost never provided counselors or social workers to help patients deal with the personal impact of illnesses on their lives and their family interactions. The separation between the emotional and the medical was stark. Medical staff dealt with medical problems affecting organs, but not the people attached to them. At regular appointments, physicians took little notice of the stretch marks. Nobody discussed them with Ellen.

Finally, Ellen told me, she brought up the subject, asking one of her surgeons directly about the stretch marks. She assumed that they were temporary and would soon fade, and wanted to know when that would happen.

"When will these go away?" she asked, drawing a finger down one of the long stretch marks inside her arm. The doctor, whom she knew well by then, seemed genuinely startled at her question, as if he were not talking to a person experiencing the aftermath of a years-long traumatic event, but a collection of body parts disassociated with feelings, emotions, and anxieties.

"Those?" he said, peering at her, and not quite shrugging. "Oh, those will never go away."

Ellen was stunned into speechlessness. A few moments later, he swept out of the examining room with a cheery wave.

The stretch marks upset Ellen most of all, but they also horrified me. I always imagined as adults we would have careers—our mother was determined that her girls, particularly, would be able to support themselves—and I assumed we would both marry and have children, too. Would Ellen even be able to date with these marks on her body? I no longer felt guilty about being able to eat while Ellen could not. Instead, I felt guilty about my own developing body, free of marks except for freckles gained from the sun. And worst of all, I was embarrassed about the way Ellen looked.

I was deeply ashamed of my reactions. *At least*, I thought, *the marks didn't affect her face, with its now-rosy cheeks, her laughing eyes, her smile with its white, even teeth, or her beautiful, thick, auburn hair.* With a long-sleeved shirt, and pants, nobody would know.

But why should it matter? I argued with myself. *Why is body image so important, especially for a girl? Would her stretch marks haunt us as much if she were male? Would they matter? And in any event, did looks matter more than kindness, more than the contributions of Ellen's mind, her faith, her heart?* Of course not.

The stretch marks made me think about Tommy Johnson, a fixture in Newcott, the most outgoing person anyone knew. When Tommy was ten, he peered inside one of his father's gasoline containers. He opened the top and looked in. Seeing nothing in the darkness, he decided he needed a light.

He lit a match.

The resulting explosion ripped most of his face and ears off, and only by a tilt of his head did Tommy somehow manage to save his eyes.

But he would undergo ten years of operations before little children, seeing him on the street, did not react by screaming and running away. Tommy could not hide his scars, but they made him determined to accept himself, his life. He refused to hide. He attended college and married a beautiful woman.

By the time I knew him, he was middle-aged. He still had bulbous ears and scar tissue layered over his face. His lips always looked strange, but he was warm and friendly, especially with kids, and he would get down at their level and speak softly to them with an attentiveness, a reassurance, that sparked their trust and made them forget his looks.

Everyone knew Tommy, and everyone liked him. His looks didn't matter. He had overcome his scars by dint of his determination and personality. He was proof that any looks could be overcome. Still, it seemed to me as though having an ugly face, or an unattractive body, was easier for a male than a female. For example, Tommy's scarred head held the thinnest patches of hair, but many men lost their hair as they aged. Had he been a woman, I knew his looks would have been more of an impediment.

Ellen's face was still beautiful, and yet the stretch marks writhed across her body out of sight and underneath her clothes from the armpits down. I brought the stretch marks up with my mother one day, telling her how awful I thought they looked and how they troubled me. Mom's reaction was fierce and immediate.

"I can't—*I won't*—worry about them," she erupted. I was startled; she was so rarely angry, but now I saw her unfettered rage about Ellen's situation for the first time, the white-hot fury that, for all I knew, she felt for years.

"Ellen. Is. Alive," she said, hissing every word for emphasis. "She is *alive*. Do you hear me? We can't—*I can't*—give her more than that. Anything else comes second. Don't *bother* me about her stretch marks."

I understood. Mom had given everything she could to help Ellen, even to the point of giving up a body part. And I was also aware that the transplant was a medical breakthrough. If Ellen's kidney had failed even a decade earlier, she would have died. If we lived in nearly any other state other than New York when our insurance stopped paying medical bills, she would have died, or we would have gone bankrupt trying to pay the endless invoices.

I weighed all this as the stretch marks got longer and wider. But Ellen rarely discussed the subject, or her feelings about them with me. I never talked about them again to my mother.

I wish I had told her the truth: That they were the scars of a warrior. Her strength and spirit meant so much more than the lines on her body.

Ellen wore shirts with long sleeves, even to swim. I wish I had encouraged her to wear a normal bathing suit if she wanted and to say to hell with the reaction of anyone else. Allowing strangers to make her feel self-conscious was an exercise in absurdity, a concession to ignorant people who didn't know better than to gape.

Years later, Ellen made a close friend, Rosanne Hartman, who rented an apartment on Anderson Place. She was appalled when Ellen told her that she wore long-sleeved shirts in the swimming pool, and with bluntness and the passionate conviction of truth, told her to just let people stare. "It was *their* problem," she said, not Ellen's.

I heard the joy in Ellen's voice when she repeated what Rosanne had said. That support gave her the permission she needed to shed the heavy shirt and don a normal bathing suit in the pool. Rosanne said what I should have, but didn't.

Instead, I wanted, for the first time, to be separate from Ellen. I longed to be in a normal family, free of tubes, syringes, needles, pills, hospitals, worries. I wanted to escape.

At the very moment I dreamed of separation, Ellen became clingy. Perhaps because she, too, was disappointed. She might have also thought that life would turn back to a time before she ever became ill. Perhaps she wanted to make up for all those weeks and months of hospital stays when I was no closer than the parking lot, five stories below.

Whatever I did, Ellen wanted to do. Wherever I went, Ellen wanted to be there, too. Yet, the two areas of my life where I wanted her presence, where I despaired, she couldn't help me.

She couldn't be with me in eighth grade, where I wished she could help defend me against bullies.

And she couldn't help me when I couldn't stop thinking about being raped.

CHAPTER 33

AREN'T GIRLS EQUAL?

DURING THAT DIFFICULT TIME, SOME WONDERFUL PERSON GAVE ME MAYA Angelou's magnificent autobiography, *I Know Why the Caged Bird Sings.* Something had happened to her during her childhood that was similar to what had happened to me, I thought, as I read the book over and over. Yet she survived to triumph, overcoming obstacles of racism, segregation, and fear that I had never come close to experiencing. It gave me hope.

I never dreamed that, years later, I would spend a memorable afternoon deep in conversation with Angelou, her warmth and wisdom so like the long-remembered tone of her book. That kind of shining future was so far beyond the struggle of the moment.

Yet, to my thirteen-year-old self, Angelou's writing and example showed me that hard times could be temporary. That was enough for most days.

But not all. There were days when I couldn't get the assault out of my head, going over and over the details nonstop, and sinking deeper into depression.

On top of the rumination, school continued to be a daily dread. When I left the house, the only question was how bad the bullying would be that day.

The behavior of a few boys wasn't just antipathy toward me, I thought, but toward all girls in general. In 1970, the women's movement was sweeping the nation. At home, my mother, my sisters, and I took feminism seriously even if it had yet to make serious inroads in the patriarchal culture of blue-collar Buffalo. The outnumbered men at home were smart enough to nod and flee most discussions.

My mother couldn't agree more with women's equality.

"It was high time that women were paid equally and got the respect they deserved," she said, and we girls talked about it with an eager eye toward our own futures.

My sister Claudia had entered D'Youville College by then, working two jobs to pay for tuition. Somehow, she found time to attend the occasional meeting of the National Organization for Women, and one day brought home Ashley Montagu's *The Natural Superiority of Women*.

I read the book eagerly. The opening sentences in the second chapter articulated my own simmering feelings:

> *"Why is it that, in most of the cultures in which we have any knowledge, women are considered to be a sort of lower being, a creature human enough, but not quite so human as the male, certainly not as wise nor as intelligent; and lacking in most of the capacities and abilities with which the male is so plentifully endowed? How is it come about that women have occupied a position of subjugation in almost all the cultures of which we have any knowledge?"*

The book sparked a solemn promise to myself: I would never, ever take a man's name in the event I got married. I realized that I *had* a man's name—my father's. But I liked the name Casey, and it infuriated me that when women got married their identity disappeared. A woman was no longer "Jane Jones," if she married "John Smith." She became "Mrs. John Smith." That's the way married women were referred to in the pages of the newspapers delivered to our home every day. You could see it in one article after another. The moment a woman said, "I do," she became a mere appendage. Well, not for me, I decided. It was a good test; if a man was miffed that I wouldn't take his name, he wouldn't be right for me anyway.

The book made me examine not just the bullying I experienced at school, but the general contempt on the playground I observed whenever the abilities of women or girls were discussed. One boy was adamant.

"The fact that so few women did anything in history proves their inferiority," he said.

Men were replete with accomplishments, the implication being that if women were capable, they would be too. Yet, the stories of women in history who had done amazing things were ignored in our classrooms. And males seemed oblivious to the fact that women could accomplish far more if they did not face barriers in the form of discriminatory laws, biased religious traditions, and restrictive societal attitudes.

It was infuriating.

My eighth-grade life was a continuation of the bullying I had experienced in lower grades, with the same two boys inflicting torment—one a follower, one the leader. Jordan was the evil genius and Axel, his ever-loyal minion, provided an audience and constant backup. Jordan would laugh at my long, black hair, my smile, my alleged smell, my intellectual inferiority, and Axel would agree and add a comment of his own. But the truly shrewd nature of Jordan's torture occurred in the random nature of its timing. I never knew when it would occur, so I was always on edge. Jordan would jeer at me during quiet moments of class when we had a substitute teacher or an instructor with little class control. He would sidle up to me and hiss invectives in the cafeteria, in the hallways, or in homeroom, but rarely alone, and always trying to win the favor of an audience. He always found a few boys to laugh or make remarks themselves. Several boys in class refused to participate, a mercy I appreciated, yet they also didn't intervene.

My mother said he did these things because he liked me, and repeatedly told me to ignore it like she had in the past. I thought her contention that when a boy likes a girl, he tries to make her life miserable was pretty close to insanity.

And the school was more concerned about the length of the girls' skirts than the boys' harassment of girls. I had no idea how to make the bullies stop.

The one bright light in eighth grade was that I landed in the same homeroom with a student I had known in second grade. Mary Teresa was more outgoing than me, with a good sense of humor. She became my one steadfast and loyal friend. She always got angry at those who taunted me, and while I was grateful that I had a friend who I could talk to and who would give me some solace from the tension at home and the teasing at school, I didn't want anyone to share my miserable isolation. I was afraid that the negative attention I received would spill over into her life, too. But Mary was made of strong stuff.

There was one area where she wouldn't follow me, however, and it involved a decision that made it even less likely that I would have more friends among the girls. Unlike every single girl in my class, I refused to be a cheerleader.

Any athletic team in school was reserved for boys alone. There was only one organized activity that girls were allowed to do in school: cheerleading.

Mary Teresa and the other girls loved cheerleading, and practice was part of the girls' gym class, along with other activities like kickball. But I refused to be a part of the ritual of leaping and shaking pom-poms. I thought it was outrageous that, to the school administration, virtually the only acceptable athletic activity for girls involved cheering on male students for engaging in sports that female students were forbidden to play.

I said as much to the gym teacher—an approachable, middle-aged woman who, in a rare moment of self-disclosure, had told me a month earlier that she was taking courses at night to finish her college degree. I told her she should finish that degree no matter what. My enthusiasm made her smile, so she was sympathetic to my objections to cheerleading. She told me to skip it, and encouraged me to dribble and shoot basketballs, which she knew I liked, while the girls practiced their cheers.

The cheers named every boy on the team and in class. I refused to cheer on my tormentors. So, I shot baskets and listened while the girls shook pom-poms, jumped, twirled, and chanted.

Jordan, Jordan, he's our man, if he can't do it, nobody can!
Axel, Axel, he's our man, if he can't do it, nobody can!

I boycotted this and every cheer. Instead, I practiced shooting baskets for a team that only existed in my head. My refusal to bond with other girls over this one shared activity increased my isolation, but for me, the price of doing otherwise was too high.

CHAPTER 34

"WRITE. JUST WRITE."

IN OUR ELEMENTARY SCHOOL WORLD, RULES RULED. ENGLISH CLASSES WERE replete with dictums.

Most written assignments came in the form of book reports. They should have been simple for me since I was constantly reading and typically read several books a month.

The more interesting books were the ones I found in our house or the cottage. I had read a racy book named *Messalina* when I was nine years old despite not understanding any of the myriad sex scenes. (The book, about the wife of the Roman Emperor Claudius, is described this way: "One of the most depraved women in all history, Messalina used her body in a game of politics until she found a man she could not destroy.") When my mother discovered that *this* was the first adult book I had chosen to read, she convulsed with laughter. She then went through the book and blotted out all the bad words with a black felt pen, a tradition that she followed for years as books became racier until it seemed as though half the paperbacks in the house were written in Morse code. Mom then gave me *A Tree Grows in Brooklyn* to read, its five hundred pages taking me a month to complete.

Yet, when it came to school book reports, I pretended I wasn't reading a thing.

Each book report required a written outline first, complete with Roman numerals and lower-case letters, titles, subtitles, all with their own rules of capitalization. If the outline was wrong, if the Roman numerals were mixed up, if you forgot to put the date in the left corner of the page or, instead, put it on the right-hand side, there would be so many points deducted that it wouldn't matter if your summary of the book was brilliant. Rules mattered. Not writing.

I hated it.

Then Mr. Pasquale arrived.

He often looked tired. No wonder. Teaching eighth-grade English at Cathedral School was his first job as an instructor while he took courses at night to finish his degree. Adolescents can smell inexperience in a teacher like hounds on the hunt, and sometimes Mr. Pasquale had to yell himself hoarse to control the inevitable chaos that erupted in his classroom.

Yet, he was also far more imaginative than teachers whose years of the daily slog of teaching had long since snuffed out enthusiasm or creativity. And Mr. Pasquale had both. His assignments were unexpected and creative. He gave us homework assignments that were free of typical rules and structure, and sometimes, when we got our work back, they had no letter grades at all, just encouragement and thoughtful comments written in the margins. His approach helped ease a kind of writing anxiety, at least for school, that I had begun to feel years earlier.

One of these unorthodox assignments changed the course of my life.

In January of 1971, he told us to bring in blank composition books. The assignment, he said, would go until the end of the school year. We were to keep a journal. We could write whatever we wanted. He told us not to worry about spelling, sentence structure, or grammar. He wouldn't grade us on that. He would just look at the journals occasionally to make sure we were doing the assignment.

"Write every day, or once a week," he said. "Your choice. Write stories, or what you see in a park, or what you thought of when you woke up in the morning."

The substance of what we wrote in the journals wouldn't matter, our teacher said. What mattered was the act of writing.

"Forget about any rules," he said. "Free yourselves from all that. Write what you feel, and what you know to be true."

We looked at each other. Everyone was confused. Forget about spelling? No rules at all? It was unlike any assignment we had ever received.

"Write. Just write."

That night, I opened the new composition book I had purchased with its blank, lined pages. The only diary I had ever read was Anne Frank's *Diary of a Young Girl*. After mulling it over, I decided to begin mine in the form of letters, too. But within a few weeks I dropped the artifice, as my initial stiffness and formality fell away.

Instead, when I came home from school, I would open the notebook and automatically begin to fill the pages. I wrote observations about Big Band music, which I loved, and how I had to keep my devotion to the music of the 1940s a secret from my Beatles-crazed classmates. I wrote how tired I was of the gray winter days; my hopes for high school; my worries about Ellen; and my dreams of travel. Often after writing, I would look at my alarm clock, thinking ten minutes had passed, and I was always surprised to see that an hour or more had gone by. No matter what mood I was in when I began to write, I felt better by the time I finished.

A blank page, I found, always listened and never interrupted. Writing became the place where I could channel all my anxieties and fears and find, if not answers, at least comfort. It became my daily meditation; my quiet place in a turning world. That simple composition notebook became the sanctuary where I contemplated all there is about who I was.

After a few weeks of constant writing, I handed in my notebook along with everybody else in class, my heart in my throat, experiencing that first rush of vulnerability that all writers feel when exposing their words to another for the first time. When Mr. Pasquale returned my notebook, I was thrilled to read what he had written in the margins, in red pen:

THESE PAGES ARE A JOY TO READ. KEEP GOING!

He didn't edit what I had written. Instead, he cheered me on.

His encouragement was life-changing. The act of near-daily writing saved my sanity. Writing a diary was the therapy I had needed for years. If the dark side of elementary school was its gauntlet of bullying, the joy of writing was its greatest gift.

Toward the end of eighth grade, in March, Mr. Pasquale announced that he was taking all of us to a play at Buffalo's Studio Arena theater. The play was *The Effects of Gamma Rays on Man-in-the-Moon Marigolds*. A real movie star, Shelley Winters, played the lead actress. Everyone was excited. Mr. Pasquale said he needed a few parents to volunteer as chaperones.

A possible plan to address the constant harassment I endured every day took shape.

I would ask my mother to be a chaperone. She was funny and kind. Heck, in our neighborhood, she was famous; the only mother anyone knew who literally gave part of her body to save her child in an operation that was still viewed as a medical miracle. I knew that my mother would dazzle my classmates. Those who bullied me would see how wonderful she was and leave me alone, if only for a few days, but possibly, I hoped, for the rest of the school year.

Her coming on this trip would be just the break I needed. I shared none of this with my mother, of course.

I asked my mother if she would chaperone our class.

"Sure," she said, absently, but without hesitation. "How nice that your teacher is taking you to a play."

CHAPTER 35

THE CAT AND THE PIT BULL

WHEN THE DAY ARRIVED, I WAS UP EARLY. THE LAST LINGERING DAYS OF WINTER had given way to a fine, early spring morning. I walked out on the porch for a few minutes, before putting on my green plaid uniform, to let in our cats from their nighttime prowls.

I saw Clara start to cross our narrow driveway. She was a tiny Tabby cat, just about a year old, gentle and affectionate, and she adored my mother, trotting after her like a dog. At odd moments, Clara would curl up on her lap, purring sleepily, while my mother read, stroking her soft fur. She was, as Mom would say, as sweet as the morning. And so small as to be nearly defenseless.

At the same moment Clara began to head toward our house, Biff, a pit bull mix that neighbors owned, saw her from across the street. I was afraid of Biff. He wasn't a dog you wanted to pet. He was rarely loose. But here he was, ambling home after some nightly escapade. He saw Clara the moment I did and stopped. Then, like a cobra, he struck, darting across the street faster than I dreamed possible. I ran down the porch steps to try to reach Clara, but Biff cornered her against the house, mauling her. She let out a screech of pain.

I screamed at Biff and threw a handful of dirt in his eyes. Startled, he stepped back for a moment and Clara tried to move, to escape, but her broken body wouldn't respond. Biff reached for her again and I flailed at him. He jumped away, and almost with a canine shrug, continued trotting down the street toward his house.

The commotion brought Mom out to the porch. When she saw Clara, she went pale. I picked up the bleeding cat as carefully as I could, and Mom brought out a small blanket in which to carry her twitching body. Clara was still alive.

"Maybe she can still be saved," Mom said, and I, barely breathing, nodded.

She ran to get her car keys, and I carefully climbed in the front seat of the station wagon, trying to move Clara as little as possible. Mom and I drove to an animal hospital about three miles away. She took Clara from me as we walked in and cradled her tiny body, whispering to her softly. The veterinarian quickly brought us to an examining room, but it was too late. Clara went limp and died in my mother's arms.

Neither of us said much driving home. Mom gripped the steering wheel so tightly I thought her fingers would leave indents. She parked in front of the house and, for a few moments, stared through the windshield, saying nothing. I felt like we were sinking.

"Don't forget, you're going to be a chaperone today," I said with a false cheerfulness. She said nothing.

"Mom? The play? Remember?" I said.

"Oh, yes," she said.

She slowly turned her head to me, as if forcing her body to remember how to move. "Right. The play."

She put the car in park, but didn't turn off the engine.

"You go on to school. I'll see you later." She paused and stared forward. "I just need to be alone for a few minutes."

Apprehensive, I walked up the stairs. When I turned around, she was gone.

By 9 a.m., all the chaperones had arrived except Mom. I insisted to Mr. Pasquale that she would arrive any minute. I knew she would be in her best brown and white dress, the one she wore for special occasions, her smile winning everyone over. The bus pulled into the parking lot and my chattering classmates began to line up, on their best behavior under the watchful eyes of their parents.

"Maura, we can't wait any longer," Mr. Pasquale said. "Something must have come up. It's OK. Maybe your mom will meet us at the theater."

"She's coming," I said, stubbornly. "I'll just wait, and get to the theater after she comes."

He nodded and said he would leave our tickets at the box office.

The minutes crawled by. The longer I waited in the quiet, empty school hallway, the more I felt on the verge of tears. The memory of the little cat's gruesome death and my mother's growing absence made my thoughts bounce between trauma and despair.

Finally, I used the office phone to call my father at work. He arrived soon after the phone call. Seeing my disappointment, he was kind, and said that maybe something had come up for my mother. He dropped me off at the theater and drove back to work.

The play would win the Pulitzer Prize a few weeks later. It features Tillie, who is trying to complete an experiment for the school science fair, despite the efforts of others to sabotage her work.

I entered the darkened theater and found a seat in the back. A moment later, Tillie's rival, Janice, began to talk about her own science project.

Janice's experiments take place on a dead cat.

"I got the cat from the A.S.P.C.A. immediately after it had been killed by a high-altitude pressure system. That explains why some of the rib bones are missing, because that method sucks the air out of the animal's lungs and ruptures all the cavities. . . . Then I boiled the cat in a sodium hydroxide solution until most of the skin pulled right off, but I had to scrape some of the grizzle off the joints with a knife.

"You have no idea how difficult it is to get right down to the bones."

In the darkness, numb and alone, I thought about Clara.

My mother apologized later. She had driven alone for hours, sobbing over the cat. Then she wondered why she was crying so much about a cat.

But I knew.

We were Clara, and life was a pit bull just waiting to shake us in its jaws.

Chapter 36

Ripping Up the Report Card

As spring unfolded, and my sadness over Clara eased, small buds of optimism began to emerge. I knew I would soon be leaving the trial of eighth grade behind.

I would go to high school in the fall of 1971, taking two buses across the city to attend the century-old Catholic school for girls that my mother had briefly attended more than thirty years before. Against all odds, she had kept her childhood vow that, if she ever had daughters, they would all attend Holy Angels Academy, the beloved school that her penurious father had allowed her to attend for only one memorable year. My sister Claudia had graduated from the school the year before. Ellen and I would be freshmen together.

Coughing up tuition money was the one financial issue over which she went toe-to-toe with my father. She successfully wrangled out of him the $500, then $600, annual tuition, although every year their pitched battles in this regard became more contentious.

I didn't get a vote, but her plans were fine by me. I knew how much my sisters loved Holy Angels, and looked forward to entering the haven of a safer, all-female environment.

As graduation approached, the bullying became downright unimpressive. I would give the mocking boys a long stare, as if saying, "Is that the best you can do?"

They were going through the motions, I sensed, with the end so close. Verbal abuse lost its sting with liberation in sight. Finally, the day before graduation, I came home with my report card in hand and a smile on my face. My marks were lackluster, but I passed.

Claudia and Ellen understood that my joy on the last day of school was mingled with relief.

"What do you want to do?" Ellen said.

"I want to rip up my report card and throw it on the convent steps," I replied.

The convent was a large stone house located next door to the school.

Claudia and Ellen looked at one another with evil grins.

Claudia helped me tear the report card in tiny little bits, especially where my name appeared, and poured the pieces in a paper bag. She and Ellen walked the two blocks with me back to the school, from which I had joyfully skipped away just a few hours before. We sprinkled the pieces of the blue-and-white report card like confetti over the convent steps and ran away, laughing.

The next day, as I assembled with my class to graduate, Sister Hildegard yanked me out of line.

"We found your report card in *pieces* all over the convent steps!" she fumed. "What is your explanation for this outrage?"

I looked at her, eyes wide and innocent. One lie after another came tripping off my tongue.

"Funny thing, I lost the report card on my way home yesterday. My goodness. Do you think someone would have been mean enough to tear it up?" I asked.

She stared at me.

"You really have no idea who did this? None?" she said, eyes narrowing.

I shrugged and shook my head.

"You must have a report card. After graduation, I insist that you return to your homeroom. I will fill out a new report card for you myself."

"How nice of you," I said, sweetly. "I'll see you right after the ceremony."

Instead, after graduation, with my life rolling out before me like a red carpet, Mary Teresa and I went to the Quaker Bonnet restaurant for hot fudge sundaes. We went our separate ways, and that fall, to different schools.

And a few months after graduation, Jordan, the boy who tormented me every day of eighth grade, called the house and asked me to go out on a date with him.

I told him I'd rather be dead and hung up.

CHAPTER 37

THE MISSING PORK CHOPS

LIKE ME, ELLEN LOOKED FORWARD TO HIGH SCHOOL. AT SOME POINT, SHE decided to just accept her scars and move on. Our handsome new uniforms of navy-blue blazers, white blouses, gray skirts, and navy-blue knee socks would hide the stretch marks, with just the back of her legs showing. Even that glimpse was enough now and then for a fellow classmate to ask me, concerned, if Ellen was okay, and if she had been in a car accident. I would always explain the source of the stretch marks, reassuring my classmates that despite appearances, they didn't hurt.

We would wear bloomers for gym class, but Ellen had a permanent medical excuse from attending. As her kidney was now located below her abdomen in front, not in back, doctors were aghast at the potential for an errant volleyball to injure the organ.

As the immediate threat of rejection receded, doctors lowered the steroid dose gradually from its whopping 200 mg a day. With a reduction in dosage, her steroid-induced diabetes disappeared.

The mood swings stayed. In her least-reasonable moments I had to remind myself that her emotions were always distorted by medication. Our mother imposed a blanket ban on fighting or arguing with Ellen because of the variety and dosage of drugs she took from the vials crowded on a small antique bureau in the bathroom. In the normal, every-day scuffle of childhood, Ellen would get a daily pass.

Yet, now that Ellen's health was no longer in a constant state of crisis, Dad's deepening alcoholism took center stage, as did the increasing dinginess of our surroundings. He continued to refuse to spend money on maintenance or repairs. Having a girlfriend, we agreed with grim sarcasm, was mighty expensive. An errant fingernail would shower paint chips from the outside of the house; our home hadn't seen a paintbrush for a decade. The porch had missing balusters that left wide, irregular gaps, like missing teeth. The railing had rotted off the front steps and its boards were becoming spongy from the relentless weather. Our genial mailman threatened to stop delivering mail unless we fixed the stairs. Floorboards on the porch loosened and decayed. Holes riddled the hallway walls and dining room ceilings. Nobody had a clue how to fix anything or how to address the overall shabbiness of the house. Instead, we improvised.

The dryer in the basement stopped working when the door wouldn't stay shut, so I propped it closed with an old broom. Dad was delighted with my solution, and the dryer stayed that way for years, broom always at the ready. The bathroom was half-finished. A contractor my mother hired in the flush of her inheritance from Aunt Lil never finished tiling drywall constructed around the tub. For fear of crumbling the plaster, nobody had been able to take a shower, ever, and my father refused to pay anyone to finish the job. We continued our weekly baths.

Soon, there was hole in the bathroom ceiling. As luck would have it, I witnessed its appearance while sitting on the toilet.

The incident occurred when I was alone in the house. I entered our only bathroom assured that, for a change, no one else would be pounding on the door telling me to hurry up. Just as I settled on the throne, a rain of plaster and dust fell on and around me. I looked up and a garbage can was sliding inexorably through the ceiling, directly above my head.

I leaped to my feet, yanking up my pants, certain that at any moment the garbage can would come crashing down. I scrambled up the steep, musty stairs to the attic, mystified how a garbage can ended up in the eaves above the bathroom.

Once I entered the attic and located the object of my potential demise, I immediately understood what had happened: Mom had been telling Dad that the roof was starting to leak and had to be replaced, an expensive job given the height of our three-story house. Instead of arranging for a repair, Dad had a better idea. He carried into the attic a spare thirty-gallon garbage can and squeezed it in between the ceiling joists directly under the leak. The can was supported only by the thin slats of wood and horsehair plaster that formed the ceiling of the bathroom.

Then he forgot about it.

The garbage can collected rainwater, filling a third of the way before it began to crash through the ceiling. It was only by luck that the heavy container stopped halfway in its descent. But I had to try to pull it out or it threatened to smash into the room below, unleashing gallons of water. I pulled as hard as I could, but it was dead weight. As I lifted the can halfway, it would slip down again, inching lower and lower into the bathroom. Finally, I wedged both feet and used the weight of my body, tilted at an angle, to yank out the can. As I pulled, the garbage can tilted, pouring some of the dirty water onto me. Grime formed from plaster dust that had poured on my head.

I went downstairs. After I washed my face, arms, and hair, I heard Ellen and Dad enter the house. Enraged, I asked him what in God's name he was thinking to put a garbage can in the attic. It had nearly killed me while I was on the toilet, I ranted.

Dad's surprise turned to amusement.

"You were taking a shit and the garbage can—at that *very moment*—started falling through the ceiling?"

He doubled up in laughter, and Ellen joined him, the two of them howling in hilarity.

I left the house and walked for hours, boiling.

As Dad's drinking escalated, Ellen finally saw what her hospital stays had hidden from her. She understood what we had been living with for years. With the transplant behind us, Dad's drinking, always bad, became the central disruption in the family. At the same time, my siblings and I were all teenagers or in our early twenties. We were becoming less willing to tolerate in silence Dad's drunkenness and his continuing affair with Brigid.

I managed the tension by writing in the journals I would keep long after eighth grade, recording pages of dialogue and describing incidents and arguments. I wrote what I saw.

Dad expected filial respect around certain occasions, notably his birthday. The year he approached his fiftieth birthday, he couldn't stop talking about the milestone he was about to reach. It really troubled him. In the run-up to his birthday, Dad became worried about two facts: Not only was he completing his fifth decade here on Earth, but he had gained weight. Despite swimming laps during his lunch hour three times a week, he tipped the scales at two hundred pounds. Instead of trying to comfort him, I wrote him a bantering poem of sly cruelty, pointing out, in rhyme, that he was not only about to be a half-century old, but also he weighed, in fact, one-tenth of a ton. He took it in good humor.

Despite his worries over getting older and being out of shape, his affair continued. He would get a phone call from Brigid with its signal—two rings and then silence. She would always hang up before one of us could get to the phone. Dad hastened to call her back from the extension in the upstairs bedroom, keeping his voice low. We looked at each other knowing what would come next.

"There's a fire in the Masten District," he said, shrugging on his coat. "I'll be late." He wouldn't come home until 3 a.m.

Dad's frustration with his life flowed like a river. It was clear who was at the root of his dissatisfaction—we were. He gave Mom less and less money to manage the house. The food he bought was the cheapest possible, some of it from what we called the "rot rack" at the supermarket—the shelves that held the soft tomatoes, the bruised bananas, and the stale bread marked down to a fraction of its retail price. When Ellen or I asked for our weekly allowance, if he dispensed money at all, he would slowly unwrap dollars from the rolls of tens and twenties that he carried. At most he would give us a dollar or two, unless we begged. An argument over money would often end the same way.

"Leeches!" Dad would shout, his face reddening. "You're all leeches!"

Then he would storm out.

My older siblings—Seamus, Tim, and Claudia—were working, and made up for his neglect by slipping Mom cash. When I needed clothes, Claudia bought them for me, including my first bra. I waited at night when Dad got home to gauge just how drunk he was. I could tell by his weaving down the narrow hallway. If he bumped into walls, I waited until he was asleep to steal as much money from him as possible and give it to Mom. But he figured out that someone was siphoning money from him. He began to hide cash in different places, thwarting my plan.

By the occasion of Dad's 51st birthday, in March of 1972, none of us were in a mood to mark the day by making gestures of respect for our father that we didn't feel. We were all fed up, and agreed that we would meet his birthday in silence.

Dad arrived home that day at 7:30 p.m. He took his coat off and hung it on the newel post beside the stairs in the front hall. After several minutes of silence, he walked to where my mother was reading in the living room.

"Nobody got me presents for my birthday."

Mom looked up, feigning surprise, and put down her book.

"Seamus didn't get you anything?"

"No!" he said, growing angry.

"Tim and the girls got you nothing?"

"No!" he snarled.

"After the beautiful presents you got for their birthday? Do you remember what you got them?"

"Um, no," he said. "Can't remember. Remind me. What did I buy the kids?"

"Nothing!" Mom snapped. "Not even a cake!"

"I must have bought something!"

"You said, and I quote, 'I can't afford it,'" Mom said.

"Well, *you* didn't get me anything, goddamn it! Can't *you* even wish me a happy birthday?" Dad shouted.

Mom stood up.

"Happy birthday, tenth of a ton. Is life better now that you're fifty-one?"

Dad took a step toward Mom, and she didn't shrink away. She looked right at him, almost daring him to take a swing. He thought the better of it, turned on his heel, grabbed his coat, and walked out, slamming the door.

He came home hours later, the house dark and quiet. I woke up, and heard him lumber downstairs, rattling pans in the kitchen. It was clear he was preparing a meal. The smell of sizzling pork chops wafted up from below. After a few minutes, I could hear the oven door open, then slam shut.

Dad came roaring up the stairs.

"Who took my pork chops?!" he shouted.

I could hear everyone begin to rouse themselves from sleep.

"Somebody took my pork chops!"

"What the hell?"

"*Now* what?"

My brothers and sisters began to awaken and react from different rooms. One by one we tumbled out of our bedrooms to stare, blankly, at our father as he screamed in the upstairs hallway.

"Your mother hid my pork chops!" he railed.

"Dad," Tim said. "You're drunk."

"No, I'm not," he said, teetering.

"Dad, go to bed," Seamus said.

Mom emerged from another bedroom.

"Casey, nobody took the goddamn pork chops. For Christ's sake, go to bed."

"I won't! You took my pork chops!"

Mom reached up and snatched his glasses from his face. He was all but blind without them.

"Casey, I've got your glasses. If you don't go to bed, I swear I'll break them in half."

She walked down the hall to his bedroom.

Seamus and Tim began to push and shove him, as he shouted and protested, toward his room. Mom slipped by them and went to Claudia's room. We could hear him yelling obscenities at Seamus and Tim as they pushed him on his bed and told him to go to sleep, emerging and shutting his bedroom door behind them.

The next day, I found the pork chops still in the frying pan in which Dad had cooked them. He had put the pan in the oven before he went up the stairs to accuse Mom of theft.

CHAPTER 38

THE BATTLE OF THE SKILLET

THE NIGHT OF THE PORK CHOPS WAS THE BEGINNING OF MONTHS OF DRUNKEN scenes after Dad would come home from a night out. One morning, he parked on our tiny front lawn, blocking the porch stairs. He was snoring behind the wheel when we emerged from the house to go to school. Other times, he would walk in the house and start shouting accusations in the hallway. My older brothers and sisters would argue with him. Mom would either try to calm him down or, exasperated, needle him with sarcastic barbs. And nobody in the house was getting enough sleep.

Finally, my brothers Seamus and Tim suggested to Mom that she consider divorce. Mom didn't think it was possible. Until 1967, New York State had the strictest divorce laws in the country. The laws recognized only adultery as grounds to dissolve a marriage and generally required eyewitness testimony. Understandably, most state residents of means who desired to end a marriage either filed for an annulment or established residency in some other state to obtain a divorce.

But in recent years, the boys told Mom, New York had finally loosened the law. The state added cruel treatment, desertion, and imprisonment as grounds for divorce. But it was still far from a simple process.

State law required one party to be at fault for the failure of the marriage even if the split was amicable. Yet, the new law was a vast improvement on the old, medieval legal stricture which since the 1700s had turned a blind eye to psychological abuse, physical assault, and financial neglect in matrimony. The process of divorce, never easy, was at least possible. Mom called a lawyer.

She had other motivations. The tension in the house was a threat to Ellen's hard-won health. Her doctors became concerned when Ellen described our father's drunken scenes at her frequent medical appointments to monitor her kidney function. They watched her blood chemistry and urinalysis carefully for signs that the turmoil was having an impact. The doctors told Mom if she needed support for a divorce, they would provide a letter to the court saying that Dad's presence was a potential liability to Ellen's full recovery.

The fights at home had an impact on Mom's health, too. Suddenly, she began to experience shortness of breath during daily moments of tension. She became visibly weaker. Mom insisted it was probably late-in-life asthma.

"Imagine me getting allergies after all these years," she joked.

But that made little sense. She would experience not just short-ness of breath, but waves of nausea. Once, when she almost passed out from not being able to breathe, Claudia insisted on driving her to the emergency room of Buffalo General Hospital, where she was admitted and hospitalized for days.

She had heart disease, and it was getting worse.

"A handful of pills is all I need," she said, and her medications were added to the bureau in the bathroom where Ellen kept her pills.

The drugs helped; for the first time in years, diuretics helped her shed the excess water retention that had always made her seem plump, and nearly overnight she slimmed down to 130 pounds on her five-foot-four-inch frame. She looked healthy and more like the pictures of her when she dated our father decades before.

Even Dad noticed. But it was too late. She told him she wanted a divorce. He replied, smugly, that she couldn't possibly file for divorce; they were Catholic.

"Casey, this isn't a theocracy," she retorted.

"No matter what you do, we will always be married in the eyes of God!" he insisted.

"Well, God isn't looking."

She knew, though, that the divorce proceedings would be easier if he cooperated. She delayed, hoping that he would come around.

Instead, the fights escalated. The antagonism in the house—coupled with the fact that most of us were teens and increasingly sarcastic— added gasoline to an already-burning blaze. This became apparent when Mom needed money to pay the pharmacy for her medication.

The costs of the drugs were not high, but weren't covered by insurance, and while the Parke Pharmacy down the street ran a tab for us, the normally understanding pharmacist was beginning to lose patience. Dad was drinking a mug of beer. He and Mom both discussed the growing bill in the living room, where I was reading. The discussion turned into prolonged negotiations.

"Casey, we have to pay down some of the total, or I won't be able to get my pills," she said.

Dad began to smile. A sly look came over his face.

"If you return to my bed, I'll give you the money," he said to my mother.

I looked up and said, "What's the problem, Dad? Isn't Brigid keeping you happy?"

He turned to me, enraged, and threw a full mug of beer in my face, the suds soaking my hair and my clothes.

"See if I'll pay tuition to send you to high school!" he snapped.

I was never much of a crier, but tears of humiliation and rage ran together with the dripping foam, as I used towels to wipe my face and dry my hair. Like hawks descending on rotting meat, everyone in the house, hearing the commotion, came down the stairs and began screaming at him.

We also suspected that Brigid egged him on in his accusations and resentment. He often seemed agitated after she called him, and unless he left quickly for a date, he would start an argument. Soon, we had confirmation that his girlfriend's intent was more than merely to have an affair.

We all knew Brigid's children. I had attended school with one of her sons. Two girls were the same ages as my brothers. One day, Seamus met June, Brigid's oldest daughter, for a drink to discuss the affair.

Her behavior was an old story to their family, June explained. Brigid was a serial philanderer. The affair with our father was her fourth in fifteen years. June, the oldest, tried to protect her younger siblings, but sooner or later, she told Seamus, they would find out. Their father was chronically passive and did nothing.

My father and Brigid had even begun to take the two youngest with them on excursions to Canada, just a few miles across the Peace Bridge from Buffalo.

"They are playing house," June said bitterly.

Seamus told her that Mom was thinking of filing for divorce. June nodded.

"That's just what my mother wants," she explained to Seamus. "But not so she could have your father. That's not her goal."

June said that her mother thrived on turmoil. She enjoyed it. As soon as our mother divorced your father, Brigid would dump him, June said. She worked to get men dependent on her—almost addicted to her. Then, as soon as the men left their wives, her mother would leave them, breaking up with them immediately. Then she would find another poor sap, and start the cycle all over again.

At least one of her former lovers had experienced a nervous breakdown in the aftermath. Another attempted suicide.

June lifted her glass of white wine and tapped it against my brother's mug of beer.

"Here's to the lovebirds," she said sarcastically. "If your mom files for divorce, well, good for her. But fasten your seat belts."

My mother soon applied for divorce, on the still-novel grounds of "cruel and unusual treatment." But divorce required a court hearing and a separation period of at least one year before severing the bonds of matrimony.

At the hearing in late December of 1972, Claudia testified against my father. The judge decreed that there were, indeed, grounds for divorce. He ruled that the one-year period of separation could begin.

But my father refused to leave the house. Mom, with no job and dependent upon him financially, felt that she couldn't force the issue. Dad tried to persuade her out of leaving the marriage. But she was adamant.

Divorce embarrassed him. His drinking got worse as he became angrier about the impending end to their twenty-four-year union.

During one argument, he threw a mug of beer at me again. The feeling of the beer coursing down my face, my hair, my chest was almost familiar, but just as humiliating and enraging as the first time. In that moment, I hated him. I couldn't wait until he was out of the house.

Finally, one spring day, he crossed a line. It was to be forever referred to as "The Battle of the Skillet."

The weather was still cool, but since the water to the cottage was turned on May 1, Mom packed our heavy sweaters and she and I left to spend the weekend. Only Claudia and Ellen were home. Dad rolled in at 4 a.m.

Although doctors had gradually reduced the powerful steroids Ellen took, the daily dose was still high. As a side effect of the drugs, one of her shoulders became unstable, dislocating from time to time without warning. She would shriek with pain and, cursing, pop the errant arm back into the shoulder. Her shoulder would be sore afterwards, and she would put her arm in a sling until it felt better. That was the case on this particular Saturday. Ellen was in the kitchen using her free hand to make a hamburger for lunch in one of our iron frying pans. Dad came downstairs, groggy from sleep, drawn by the smell of the cooking, but half-blind. Somewhere amidst his bar-hopping the night before, he had lost his glasses.

He began to follow Ellen around the kitchen. He thanked her for her thoughtfulness in making a hamburger for him, saying he couldn't wait to eat it.

"Go ahead," Ellen said.

"I know I can, *kid*," Dad sneered, reaching for a hamburger roll.

"You know, Dad, you can just go fuck yourself," Ellen snapped.

"That's virtually impossible," Dad replied.

"I forgot," Ellen said. "You save it for Brigid."

Incensed, Dad began to push Ellen around the kitchen, hitting her recently dislocated shoulder with the palm of his hand. Hearing Ellen howl in pain, Claudia rushed in, yelling, "Leave her alone, Dad!"

Dad turned from Ellen to Claudia and shoved her, too. Claudia grabbed the handle of the sizzling frying pan and swung the skillet at his head in a roundhouse punch. Grease spattered everywhere. The hamburger hit the wall, spattering the flowered wallpaper and sliding to the floor. Dad raised his arms to defend himself, but Claudia continued to pummel him with the hot frying pan, hitting him four times, burning one arm and leaving a scrape on the other.

Dad fled into the front hall and picked up the phone.

"I'm going to call the police and get you out of here," he shouted.

Then he muttered, "If I can only see without my glasses."

Claudia began to laugh.

"Hell, *I'll* dial the police for you," she retorted. "I can see the headlines now: CHILD ACCUSED OF FATHER BEATING."

Dad slammed down the phone and threw the phone book at Claudia. Claudia ducked and the thick directory just missed her, hitting the wall. Ellen heard the thud of the phone book as she was picking the hamburger up off the floor.

"Come on, Ellen, I need a witness!" Claudia yelled.

Ellen ran into the hall in time to see Dad and Claudia lunge at each other like prizefighters. Dad grabbed Claudia's right arm, but she was always left-handed and slammed him hard enough on his face that blood began to spurt out of his nose.

The bleeding stopped him. He covered his nose with one hand, with the other groped for a tissue.

"You hit me! I'm bleeding!" he said, astonished.

"Ellen, let's go," Claudia said, grabbing her car keys.

The two of them left my father, cradling his nose in the front hallway.

I was surprised to see them come walking across the lawn at the cottage and called for Mom, and they relayed what had happened. Claudia's arms were bruised blue where Dad had grabbed her. Although Claudia and Ellen joked that Dad had gotten the worst of it, I could see they were both upset. Mom listened, then slammed her fist on the table.

"That's it. He's *not* touching my babies."

Monday morning, she called her lawyer, who filed for a restraining order against Dad. He had no choice but to pack and move out of the house. He moved into a fifty-five-dollar-a-month apartment in South Buffalo's First Ward.

The day he left, Seamus changed the locks on the front door.

Soon after, Claudia enlisted in the Marine Corps. She wanted to get as far away from home as she could.

CHAPTER 39

PAYCHECKS AND POLITICS

BEFORE DEPARTING FOR MARINE CORPS BOOT CAMP, CLAUDIA TOLD ME SHE was gay. It frightened me. I didn't want her to get hurt, or vilified. I also knew that Claudia's sexual orientation could result in a dishonorable discharge. I told no one, and worried in silence.

Later, when Claudia graduated from boot camp, she told Mom. I walked into Mom's bedroom a few minutes after Claudia had told her and both were smiling. After her revelation, Claudia said, our mother didn't skip a beat.

"Honey, people fall in love with people. It doesn't matter who you love, just as long as you really love them."

Everyone hoped that the court hearing to come would award Mom alimony, but we knew it wouldn't be enough. My brothers and sisters continued to give her a portion of their wages, with Seamus, Tim, and Claudia giving the most. Claudia mailed fifty-dollar bills from boot camp.

At fifteen, I didn't have a job, and I had outgrown my childhood stint as a professional mourner. I still stayed overnight at the funeral home from time to time to answer any middle-of-the-night phone calls from hospitals with instructions for body pickups. But those occasional shifts weren't enough, and I was desperate to help my mother.

Fortunately, on the island, the son of our elderly neighbor, Grace Cohen, offered me a summer job. He would pay me $25 a week if I slept overnight in their cottage during the week. Rex would spend every weekend at the cottage with his mother, but he worried that Grace's failing eyesight would cause her to fall in the middle of the night. Even though the cottage had been in their family for forty years, he was concerned that one sleepy night, she would stumble, break a hip, and lay there without help until daylight.

I agreed, but negotiated. I told him if he paid me another $10, I would mow the front lawn every week. He accepted immediately and I had a summer job. I spent half of my first weekly check of $35 to take my mother out to dinner, then I started contributing to the household like my brothers and sisters. It was a habit that would continue with a nursing home job, which enabled me to give Mom part of my weekly wages of $75. My siblings and I hoped that our combined efforts might bring in enough to help her manage.

Staying overnight at the Cohen cottage was a different experience from sleeping on my informal sunporch bed. The place always smelled a little musty. But getting to know her was compensation worth more than money.

Her eyesight was poor, and she asked me to read to her the latest developments in the Watergate scandal from newspapers and magazines. Grace was fascinated by current events and, despite being a Republican, hated Richard Nixon with a passion. She would discuss each story with me, adding the considerable wisdom she had accrued from her nearly ninety years on the planet. Our discussions were like seminars in political analysis.

I had another motivation for attempting to understand the events unraveling on Capitol Hill. Claudia was cut off from the outside world. She and her fellow recruits in boot camp had no access to news. She asked me to summarize what was happening in my letters, so I did, sending her fat envelopes with political articles along with long letters summarizing the week's events.

The exercise increased my interest in politics and journalism. I began to notice that women reporters were making inroads from the women's sections. Elizabeth Drew's coverage of Watergate for *The New Yorker* was incomparable. I cheered on all those cool female journalists broadcasting for the then-new National Public Radio, who were hired, unbeknownst to me, not merely because they were qualified, but because so few men would accept the radio network's poor salaries. Yet, their presence made a difference. I began to think that I could, too, when I got older.

I used my little paychecks to help Mom and save money for a motor. The year before, Tropical Storm Agnes spawned huge waves in Lake Ontario and in the normally placid harbor. The storm left the *Banana Boat* shattered beyond repair and the waves sent pieces of the splintered runabout into the maw of the storm. But even before that unusual event, the *Banana Boat* had become a sad shadow of its former self, with yellow paint flaking off its side, a floating version of the dilapidated house we lived in on Anderson Place. We were back to rowing for the time being.

The cottage, bought when it was newly painted, still looked good in contrast. We could hold our heads up high there, and not be embarrassed by peeling paint. We fit in with Island society, and had the luxury of creating new routines there, both good and bad.

In the late afternoons, one of us would make dinner and Mom and I would both play a few games of rummy before I left to walk to Grace's cottage. As I shuffled the deck, Mom would make a drink. I would open a beer before I began to deal the cards. Having at least one beer at night had become a ritual. My mother paid no heed. At fifteen, I was old enough to learn how to "handle it."

Our card games were fiercely competitive, laced with alcohol and leavened with humor.

If I won, my mother would look at me, frown, and say, in mock rage, "In the interest of fair play, I insist you roll up your sleeves."

"I'm wearing a tee shirt," I would reply.

"You can't fool me. You're cheating."

"Don't be such a sore loser. You're setting a bad example."

If I won again, Mom would begin to hurl elaborate insults.

"You are a continual reminder to me that my grandparents were first cousins," she would say.

"Hah! Genetically, that would have far more impact on you than me," I said.

"That's not true," Mom would say, lighting a cigarette. "In any event, it is clear to me that you people have held me back for far too many years. If it weren't for you goddamn kids, I would be a high-class streetwalker in Miami by now."

The repartee would always end in one of us laughing.

My mother, ever the night owl, would sleep until 8:30 or 9, while I was up by 6:30, with a morning optimism that both amused and irritated her.

"If you must persist in being so goddamn cheerful all the time, the least you could do is make breakfast," she would say.

That morning meal became my specialty. After making breakfast for myself, Mom, and any guests who were staying at the cottage,

I would head down to the beach, notebook under my arm. I would settle back on a sun-bleached log, listen to the waves pounding like the heartbeat of summer, and write.

Writing had become to me as necessary as breathing. I would fill notebook after notebook about my hopes for the future, conversations that I had with neighbors, how much I missed my sister Claudia and how Ellen, shocked to have survived her childhood, felt increasingly frustrated.

CHAPTER 40

THE COST OF GIVING

DECEMBER OF 1973, ELLEN WOULD TURN EIGHTEEN AND WOULD BE A JUNIOR in high school because of the years of her illness. While I loved our high school, she chafed at its rules.

Ellen was the oldest in our class by two years. Her age made her impatient with the restrictions of a Catholic high school. But her experiences did, too. She had endured years of following medical directives whether or not she wanted to. Now she was clearly irritated with more rules.

Her frustration found an outlet in hijinks. The nuns never found out that she was the one to drape a sign on the life-sized statue of the Archangel Gabriel that dominated the second floor. The angel had one hand on the head of a statue of a smiling child; the angel's other hand was raised, forefinger pointing heavenward. The sign Ellen hung said: BARKEEP, GET ME ONE MORE BEER FOR THE KID.

Ellen did get in trouble when, over the school loudspeaker, she invited students to join the chess club if they were having problems mating. A year after the transplant, in September of 1971, Ellen made tee-shirts that said: A YEAR OF WASTE.

Looking forward to Mom's birthday in August, Ellen began to insist that, since she had Mom's kidney, she, too, should receive birthday presents on August 19.

Ellen still didn't have a driver's license. When she got restless in the city and decided to stay with Mom and me at the cottage, she often couldn't get a ride to Newcott. Sometimes, she rode a bike the forty miles between the city and the Island, which would have seemed impossible when her disease had reduced her to an exhausted wraith. She would arrive, tanned, sweating, and smiling. Her robust health was a miracle.

Ellen only wanted to practice one sport: rowing. She continued to be outraged that she couldn't row at the West Side Rowing Club like our brothers. I thought her ambition to become an oarsman was a waste of time. Yes, everyone knew that just across the Niagara River, in Ontario, rowing was open to women.

Not so in Buffalo. The West Side Rowing Club had never allowed women to join since its founding in 1912. Members called many of those who ran the club the "old boys" with affection, but to me, the nickname reflected their attitudes, stuck in the past. The club had even sent a crew to the 1936 Olympics. Even so, it was hard to imagine women ever rowing with "WSRC" on their shirts as they feathered the oars in competition.

"Ellen, they will never change," I would say, shaking my head.

As Ellen grew in strength, Mom grew weaker.

For years, after getting groceries in town, Mom and I would pause to take a walk through an old cemetery located at the outskirts of the village of Newcott, admiring the trilliums growing beneath towering maple trees and reading inscriptions on tombstones.

But now Mom had less energy for such walks. Instead, we drove by the cemetery and parked near a single heart-shaped grave we always used to visit with the inscription OUR LITTLE MABEL. Mom would watch from the car as I pulled weeds and brushed off any errant twigs that had fallen around the small stone engraved with its three-word spasm of grief. Afterward, I would unload the groceries from the boat, trotting up and down the Mount Everest of our stairs while Mom walked up a few steps, rested, then walked up a few more.

After we had dinner and Mom rested, she and I would often walk a few cottages away to watch the sun setting over Lake Ontario. We joked it was better than TV, which Mom had exiled from the cottage the moment the Watergate hearings ended.

Once in a while she would amble, slowly, to visit other neighbors. I would match my mother's steps, slowing down my own and putting an arm around her shoulders. She would put an arm around my waist in return and insist that she liked to take life slowly.

"Why rush?" she would say, and I was fooled into believing that her plodding pace was a choice.

The pinnacle of the season was the end of every August, when Island residents gathered to mark the end of another summer and to gird us all for the winter to come. Everyone relished the last languid days, as the pervasive sense they were almost over began to set in.

During a combination potluck dinner and barbecue, residents always made a point to honor the oldest of the Island inhabitants. After all, who knew what the next year would bring?

CHAPTER 41

THE DIVORCE

THE 1973 COURT HEARING THAT DISSOLVED MY PARENT'S MARRIAGE OF twenty-four years and nine months felt as swift as an executioner's axe. I wrote in my journal, "As of November 1st, WE were officially divorced, joy of joys!" The dissolution took place on the Feast of All Saints; too bad it didn't occur on Halloween, my mother wisecracked.

We scanned the newspapers every day looking for the official announcement under the section reserved for court filings. We didn't have long to wait. There it was, under "Marital Actions, Divorces" on November 11, in small but clear type: JANE CASEY, OF 145 ANDERSON PLACE, FROM JAMES FRANCIS CASEY. Mom bought a half dozen copies of the *Courier Express*, the morning daily. Using scissors, she carefully cut out the announcement in each copy of the paper and gleefully pasted them in Christmas Cards.

"I know your father. He'll keep this a secret. He won't tell anyone, especially his sisters," she said.

The court granted Mom alimony of about $110 a week, which included $60 for her and child support of $50—$25 each for Ellen and me. Amounting to $5,720 a year, when poverty level for a family of four was around $5,000, it was barely enough.

Mom wanted to show us that life would be better now. She made a few subtle decisions that were outwardly small, but made a difference. The divorce, far from being the terrible burden on children that popular culture warned about, felt liberating.

She began to buy butter instead of margarine. Butter was so much more expensive than margarine that we thought only rich people could afford it. I was shocked when she brought a pound home from the store.

Next, she banished powdered milk from our lives and bought whole milk instead. It was a relief not to have to mix water with milk powder that never completely dissolved. Whole milk didn't have white powdery lumps floating on top that I had always gagged down.

The third change wasn't culinary. Mom began to order the Sunday *New York Times*. Buffalo, eight hours from New York City, was too distant from the newspaper's West 43rd Street headquarters to get any but the earliest edition, printed Saturday evening. The newspapers weren't delivered to Buffalo homes, either. To obtain a *Sunday Times*, you had to reserve one from a local store.

One such store, a coffee shop, had opened a block away. I would stand in line on Sunday mornings to pay for the newspaper. As I carried it home, I would breathe in the smell of ink, marvel at its heft, and look forward to reading stories all week long. I loved the *Courier Express* and dreamed of writing for it someday. But the *Sunday Times* was a constant revelation. The depth of its stories awed me. We argued over who would get to be first to read the book review, the Sunday magazine, or the opinion page.

My mother seemed happier than I had remembered in years. She began to make our lunches the night before for us to take to school. She always used a red felt pen to draw a heart onto the shell of the hard-boiled eggs before slipping them into the brown paper bags that held sandwiches and, perhaps, a few grapes. Our friends noticed and at lunch would peer into our bags, looking for the imprinted eggs. Mom returned to her old habit of singing arias in the kitchen. Hearing her one day, I asked her if she liked being single again. She laughed a little, and then said, softly, "I love it."

Soon after the divorce notice appeared, I saw Brigid's daughter June at the Jewish Center pool, swimming long, graceful laps. She saw me and swam to the side of the pool, removing her goggles.

"I saw in the paper that your mother finally did it. She divorced your dad. I'm happy for you," June said.

She looked up at me from the side of the pool with a little smile.

"Of course," she continued, "I didn't need the newspaper to know what happened."

"What do you mean?" I said.

"My mother left your father in the dust," June said. "She's already dating another poor bastard."

With a wave of her hand, she continued swimming laps.

CHAPTER 42

MONEY

IN THE MONTHS AFTER THE DIVORCE, DAD VIEWED THE SHARDS OF HIS LIFE FROM a tiny apartment in the Old First Ward, an area crisscrossed by railroad tracks, with small houses clustered within sight of the towering grain mills that were the sentinels of the waterfront. The industrial South Buffalo neighborhood was far from his lace-curtain Irish beginnings just a few miles away. Brigid had left him, his wife divorced him, and we, his children, were deeply antagonistic toward him.

Despite his isolation, he paid my mother alimony on time, and continued dribbling out money to us for allowances or any extras that we needed—a little money here, a little there.

To me, it quickly became clear that money was power.

My mother didn't have power because, with so many kids in so few years, she never had the time to work. Now that we were all growing up, she didn't have the health to get a job. Her experiences made her even more of a feminist. She saw how relying upon the strength of a marriage rather than education and a career had made her vulnerable. She pushed me and my sisters.

"Get a good education. Find a satisfying career," she said, over and over.

"If you end up getting married and having kids, and want to stay home with them, that's just fine," she would say. "But if you don't enter marriage with a way to have your own career, you will always be dependent on someone else. Look at what happened to me."

"If you get married and your husband isn't good to you, you ditch the dog. DITCH THE DOG," she would repeat. "If you have a degree, you'll be able to make your own way."

Yet, even though my parents were divorced, we still relied upon our father.

I avoided asking Dad for money, resenting the last vestige of control he still possessed over me. When I absolutely had to ask him for money, I felt like a serf, waiting for the coin of the realm. So, I mostly relied on my savings from working during the summer, then, during the school year.

Ellen didn't have a job, though, and her attitude was different. She saw the endless dance of extracting money from our father as an amusing game. Ellen would peck at him like a chicken. She would ask him for money every single chance she got with a relentlessness that awed me.

"Dad, I need ten dollars."

"I don't have it."

"Please. Please. I really need it. You got paid today. I need $10."

"Jesus, Ellen. What do you need it for?"

"I need some art supplies for school. Dad, I need it. You've got it. I know you do. Come on, Dad."

"Ellen, I told you, I don't have it. Will you stop?"

"Yes, you do, Dad. You have it. I know you do. Eight dollars. I'll manage with eight dollars. Come on, Dad, you can do it."

"Goddammit, Ellen, I'm telling you, I have bills to pay. Stop. All right, then. Three. Three dollars."

"Aw, Dad, you know you can do better. Five bucks, Dad. Five dollars. It's not enough, but I'll manage. Come on, Dad. Please?"

Finally, my father would roar, "Ellen! You nickel and dime me to *death*!"

But he would always hand her some cash—never as much as she had asked for, which is why she always asked for more than she needed. Later, she would laugh about it.

While his income gave him continued power over us, the divorce, Mom said, made him examine his own life and the consequences of his actions.

I found it hard to care.

"If I never see him again, it wouldn't matter," I told her.

Mom was more sympathetic.

"He blew it," she would say, but without rancor. She wasn't bitter. There was no question of them getting back together again, yet she needed his cooperation in paying alimony and child support.

After his initial shock, Dad, Catholic to the bone, could not deny the damage he had done. He felt guilty. When he came to the house, he rarely smelled of alcohol. He was serious and calm. Gone were the shouted accusations, the drunken scenes. His remorse ensured that he never missed an alimony payment. He also paid the fifty-seven-dollar-a-month mortgage separately and gave Mom money to pay the heat bill during cold months—always the biggest utility bill during Buffalo's relentless winters.

Instead of mailing a check, he stopped by the house regularly to give Mom her alimony. In February, he asked Mom out to dinner for what would have been their twenty-fifth wedding anniversary.

Mom laughed.

"Casey, we are divorced! Have you noticed?"

"Not in the eyes of God," Dad said. "In the Catholic Church, we are still married."

"I keep telling you, God isn't looking," she replied.

"Let's go out anyway. Just for old time's sake," Dad coaxed. "We'll go to the Cloister."

The Cloister—with its crystal chandeliers, its silent, attentive wait staff, and its elegant and expensive menu—was the finest restaurant in Buffalo.

My mother couldn't resist.

When they sat down to dinner, a graying, dignified waiter approached to tell them the specials in a soft voice. Startled, both my parents recognized him, but not by name.

He was the same man who had waited on them when they went out to dinner after announcing their engagement in 1948. They had come full circle.

What mom noticed the most was not just that their "anniversary" dinner cost $100, but that Dad paid for it without complaining. We were all surprised. We shouldn't have been. It was the beginning of his occasional attempts to win back my mother.

She was amused by his attention. She might have also thought that if he had a glimmer of hope for a reconciliation, he would continue to pay alimony and other bills without complaint.

One of the biggest bills was our tuition, and every September, I looked forward to school with a mix of anticipation and dread. I never knew whether Dad had paid our tuition for the previous year and always feared that he would stop paying entirely for Ellen and me, thus forcing us to drop out.

Holy Angels Academy was academically challenging, and yet the academic competition was tempered by the kindness of teachers and classmates alike. The school had patient and even brilliant instructors, a mix of laypeople and sisters. But most important, its atmosphere was emotionally supportive. After the gauntlet of bullying I experienced in elementary school, high school was a warm embrace.

Dad hated paying the tuition. But the principal made short work of Dad's reluctance. Every September she would call Dad at work to tell him to pay up in person before she had to send us home. Every September, Dad meekly appeared at school with a check.

He wasn't about to argue with clergy. They represented the Church to him. More important, they were on our side.

CHAPTER 43

COACH, CHEERLEADER, OPTIMIST

THE NUNS WHO TAUGHT US WERE LIKE A BRANCH OF THE CIA. THEY HAD informants everywhere. They knew about Dad's drinking, but they never let on to us that they knew about our home life. They also understood Ellen's medical history and never penalized her for handing in late assignments.

The nuns also intervened in my mother's academic ambitions for Ellen. Every student at the school had to take at least one three-year course of study in advanced subjects and languages besides the core subjects of history, English, basic sciences, and math.

Mom didn't believe a person was fully educated without being steeped in the mystery and beauty of Latin, which she could read effortlessly. If Ellen and I wanted to take three or even four years of math and science, that was up to us, but she was determined for us to learn the language that she had spent five years—three in high school and two in college—reading and enjoying.

But the principal pushed back. She insisted that Ellen have an easier course of study given the aftermath of the transplant and the wide variety of drugs she took. Ellen's struggles, psychological and physical, had become normal to our family, but to an outsider, her challenges were formidable. The school insisted that Ellen choose art as her three-year course of study—intellectually easier and one in which Ellen's high doses of steroids would have less of an impact.

Surprising all of us, Mom acquiesced. Ellen took art; I took Latin.

Where my mother saw beauty in the language, I experienced it as a daily torment. I never got the hang of diagramming sentences to learn grammar in elementary school. Since that was the only way school taught how to identify parts of speech, Latin, with its backward sentences, was a constant puzzle. I guessed my way through every test.

The climax of my nightmare, I knew, would be the Latin Regents exam after three years of study. I couldn't get a Regents Diploma without passing this exam, and I knew my mother expected me to pass. That meant I had to get at least a 66.

That June afternoon, when I sat to take the test, my hands felt clammy. I was nervous. I unsealed the exam and read over the questions.

I nearly burst out laughing. I expected the entire test to consist of translating Latin like previous exams. But it wasn't. Nearly half the test involved Roman history and mythology. We had rarely discussed either topic in Latin class, but I knew all about both, starting with reading picture books about those subjects when I was small. Everyone in my family could reel off the name of the Greek gods and their Roman equivalents.

My brother Tim loved ancient history and mythology so much that he never shut up about it. Thanking God for my obsessed brother and the tattered children's book still on the living room bookshelf, *The Golden Treasury of Myths and Legends*, I zipped through the questions. In the end, I got an 81, owing a burnt sacrifice to all the gods who helped me escape Latin after three non-comprehending years.

The Regents exam tradition in New York State extended to its decades-old Regents Scholarship Exam, open to any high school senior. Achieving a certain score would win a student a four-year scholarship to college. But the award was far more prestigious than the $1,000 scholarship. Those who won would have their names printed in the newspaper.

I dreamed about winning a Regents Scholarship, wistfully, knowing it was really beyond me. But I hadn't counted on the determination of one teacher. Sister Mary Kathleen Duggan was a combination drill sergeant, cheerleader, optimist, and guardian angel. When she wasn't teaching at Holy Angels, she taught at D'Youville College. In either place, she never met a negative thought in one of her students that she didn't try to exorcise.

Sister Kathleen had a broad smile and often poked fun at herself, referring to her English doctoral thesis on the writing of Milton as a cure for insomnia. While she had a good sense of humor, she was no pushover. When FBI agents came snooping around D'Youville during the Vietnam War and demanded the files of a student involved in the protest movement, Sister Kathleen not only refused, but insisted that the agents leave campus immediately and not return. They obeyed.

We students rarely saw her steel, but she awed us, nonetheless.

She recited *Beowolf* in Old English. She created an innovative course on the history of American cinema. She used movies to point out the changing societal view of women's roles, from the adventurous and resourceful female lead in *The Perils of Pauline* in 1914 to the fainting damsels of the 1930s. She took pains to emphasize the shameful glorification of racism in films, showing us the 1915 movie *Birth of a Nation,* and taught how it shaped attitudes and fed the rise of bigotry and the Ku Klux Klan. She challenged us to question what we saw on screen and in life.

When the school asked Sister Kathleen to teach Advanced Placement English in my senior year, she agreed upon one condition: that the course be open to anyone, regardless of grades. The principal consented. I signed up.

An even dozen seniors showed up for the first class. We were a mixed group. About half had the highest grade point averages in school. Then there were me and a few others with average marks. Sister Kathleen surveyed us, tucked a lock of her gray hair under her short, black veil, and smiled broadly. She announced that for the first five weeks of the class, she would not teach the normal curriculum. That would take a back seat to a far more important task.

We looked bewildered. She laughed.

"Ladies. No matter what your grades have been so far, I assure you: Every one of you is brilliant and will do great things."

She paused.

"Every single member of this class will win a Regents scholarship for college this year. The exam is in five weeks. *That* is what we will spend each class preparing for. English can wait."

My heart leapt. I wanted a scholarship more than anything. Not just for the money to attend college, but for a sign that I showed potential in *something.*

Sister Kathleen became a mix of happy warrior and demanding coach as we pored over old scholarship tests. Her belief in us was infectious. Where we looked in the mirror and saw limp hair or pimples, breasts too small or too large, bodies too thin or too fat, where we had fears and discouragement, she saw only shining possibilities.

Inspired, I studied during breaks at my nurse's aide job and at home after I returned at night. Ellen refused to take the test. She insisted that she wasn't going to attend college.

"You'll go when the time comes," Mom said, and put off that fight to another day.

The day of the exam, I left without Ellen, filled with both hope and trepidation. It was as difficult as I feared, but I kept hearing Sister Kathleen's encouraging messages in my head, sweet staccato notes that played over and over, drowning out my doubts:

"You can do this. You will do wonderful things in your life. You have so much to look forward to! The scholarship will be just the beginning."

Her torrent of praise for a time melted away any negative messages that I had been telling myself for seventeen years.

In the end, ten out of the dozen students in the class won Regents Scholarships—including me. I had hung on by my fingernails, winning a scholarship by three points.

On hearing the news, Sister Kathleen's Cheshire-cat grin was broader than ever. Some in class would have scored well on the exam and won scholarships without her help, but I knew it was her unerring confidence that carried me across the finish line.

To outward appearances, the scholarship was not momentous, yet it stunned me. My elementary school had labeled me as below-average academically. I had nearly failed sixth grade. In seventh grade, the school experimented with tracking students academically. I landed in the remedial group with other huddled masses. Other students casually referred to me and others as belonging to "the dummies" group, And yet, here I was, five years later, a scholarship winner. It was clear, right there, in the pages of both our daily newspapers. And the names of my childhood tormentors were nowhere to be found. If I could do this one thing, so against the odds, what else was possible?

Ellen, however, took a downward turn and began to flounder. Our high school guidance counselor, hapless Sister Rebecca, told her, bluntly, that she would never get into college, pointing out that her grades put her dead last in our class of seventy-five girls— yet another blow to Ellen's self-image.

In autumn of senior year, Sister Kathleen presided over study hall when a group of seniors, Ellen and I among them, set aside our books. We began to tell her about our frustrations with the guidance counselor's tendency to focus all her energy and advice on straight-A students who didn't need her help getting to college. Ellen spoke up, suddenly. I could see she was upset.

"Sister Kathleen, she told me that I would never get into college."

As I watched, horrified, my sister, who hadn't wept after losing her eye, having her kidneys removed, and who faced death calmly, began to cry. She wept uncontrollably, in front of everyone, big tears rolling down her cheeks.

"Ellen," Sister Kathleen said, getting up and swiftly crossing the room. "Ellen, listen to me. *You can go to any college you want to. You tell me where you want to go, and you will go there. I promise.*"

Ellen's crying eased, and she nodded, comforted.

Sister Kathleen looked around the room.

"I'll talk with Sister Rebecca."

I believed her. But I'm not sure Ellen did.

Ellen, who never listened to doctors' grim prognoses, found it hard to feel optimistic about applying to college when she was getting so many bad grades. The principal had been correct: the steroids she took interfered with her ability to concentrate. More to the point, the trauma she had endured in her short life also formed a barrier to her doing well in school, one that we, her family, blithely ignored. We collectively assumed that the bad old days were in the past and that Ellen should just move on.

Easy for us to say.

CHAPTER 44

GASPING FOR AIR

OUR FAMILY REMAINED CLUELESS ABOUT THE IMPACT OF THE TRAUMA ELLEN HAD endured for years.

She became ever more restless and moody, and snapped at us frequently. What was obnoxious behavior in another might have easily sparked a confrontation, but we usually ignored it, as our mother had drilled into us. Nobody asked her what was wrong. Mom and I chalked it up to medication, and Ellen usually got a pass. One night, though, tension erupted into the open. I walked into the tail end of an argument.

"It's high time you got a job and contributed like everyone else is in this house!" Seamus said, his voice rising.

"So, are you the boss now, Seamus? Really? You run the family now?" Ellen said.

"Well, somebody needs to!" Seamus shouted.

"Who do you think you are?" Ellen yelled back.

"What the hell is going on?" I said. "Seamus, what are you getting at?"

"Who asked you to butt in?" Seamus said, now turning on me.

"Mind your own goddamn business, Maura!" Ellen retorted.

Seamus threw up his hands in the air and walked out as Ellen ran upstairs to her room. I was left in the front hall, bewildered, but somehow not surprised at what had just transpired.

No wonder that Ellen felt rudderless. For years, the entire family's common goal was centered on one thing: helping her survive. After the kidney transplant, it was as if we—and she—expected everything to go back to normal. About the only break we gave her was to excuse her mood swings, but in every other way, the family expected her to be just like everyone else.

Which was, of course, impossible.

Ellen's life would never return to anything resembling normal. She had been through too much. Her body and memories bore scars of her ordeal.

She would always be overweight for her height. The stretch marks gradually turned more pink than scarlet, but remained. She still struggled with insomnia and mood swings.

And she grasped the implications of being on high doses of steroids for years. Ellen told me later that she feared that she would someday develop cancer from all the drugs she had been on. She always assumed that she would not live long, and that if she saw forty, she would be lucky.

Ellen didn't get any outside psychological help. None of us did. She needed it for what she had been through. Left unspoken was the effect of her four-year ordeal, and continuing struggle post-transplant, on all the rest of us. Voicing the negative impact of what her illness had done to us, to me, seemed impossibly selfish.

I never said words aloud that I nevertheless thought—that when Ellen became ill, her disease attacked not only her, but the entire family. Our collective façade might have been cheerful in the face of troubles, but I often felt her illness had destroyed my childhood. I rarely contemplated the impact of the disease on the rest of my siblings or my parent's marriage. Yet I knew that outside help was out of the question, even when my mother's "leave 'em laughing" philosophy inevitably fell short.

Instead, in the aftermath, several of us once again turned to the family salve. Alcohol remained the beloved ninth member of the family, present every day, the center of mourning and celebrations alike.

We lived around the corner from a liquor store, about three hundred feet from our front porch. My family helped the owner pay his mortgage. When Claudia graduated from boot camp in 1973, we rejoiced in her accomplishment in the usual way: We drank. A lot. We opened so many bottles of cheap Champagne on our front porch that the next day our tiny patch of lawn was littered with corks. I was fifteen.

After I took the dreaded Latin Regents exam, my mother met me at the door when I returned home and handed me a chilled six-pack of Champale, a sparkling malt liquor popular in the 1970s.

"Have a drink," she said. "You can either drown your sorrows or celebrate!" Celebrate I did. I was sixteen.

The day I was told that I won a Regents scholarship, I was scheduled for work and so my celebration started when I came home at 10:30 p.m. I went to bed happily drunk at 1 a.m. I had just turned seventeen.

Alcohol was the mainstay of my family. It was the center of Irish-American culture as I experienced it, and the culture of Buffalo. The bars in the city were open until 4 a.m. The legal drinking age was eighteen. But waiting until it was legal to drink never occurred to us. The idea of not drinking regularly—and by the time I was nineteen, not having a drink every single day—was not merely foreign to me. I saw abstinence as akin to a mental illness. I held two contradictory attitudes at the same time: Like the rest of the family, I condemned my father's drinking, but was entirely blind to what alcohol might do to me—or to us.

Denial, that pillar of alcoholism, often affects the family as much as it does an alcoholic who refuses to admit the destruction his actions cause. I joked about the saying, "If you drink, you die. If you don't drink, you die. So, it's better to drink." I never thought the dark side of drinking could affect me. Instead, as I looked forward to graduation, I felt only optimism.

My mother was triumphant as Ellen and I graduated from high school on that perfect June evening in 1975. She had been true to her vow made forty years before, when her father's penury forced her to leave Holy Angels after one year. All four girls attended and graduated.

Nearly all of my classmates went to college, some to prestigious schools like Georgetown. I envied them. The only college that had accepted my average grades was Buffalo State. I would go no farther away to college than the ten minutes it would take me to ride my bike a mile and a half down Elmwood Avenue.

I was lucky to live during an era when the state and federal governments believed that helping low-income students attend college was a good investment. New York State gave generous grants to lower-income college students and had one of the largest public systems of colleges in the world, second only to mainland China. I knew it would cost me next to nothing to attend.

Yet, Ellen still refused to apply to college.

After a huge argument that September, Mom told Ellen that if she didn't go to college, she had to get a job. She did, in the kitchen of Millard Fillmore Hospital, one of the few area hospitals in which she had never been treated during her illness. It was an awful job, with endless dishes and silverware to wash from conveyer belts that whisked trays in from the dining room. Most of her co-workers were mentally handicapped, but strong, efficient, and twice as fast as she was. She came home every day discouraged and exhausted.

Mom was unsympathetic.

"Get used to it," she told Ellen. "This is your future if you don't get a degree."

After a month of grueling shifts, Ellen filled out the New York State college application and agreed to go anywhere in the state college system. Sister Kathleen, true to her earlier promise, wrote a glowing recommendation, explaining away her poor marks in high school and praising her qualities of persistence, strength, and good humor.

Much to Ellen's surprise, the State University College at Potsdam accepted her. The school was three hundred miles away, less than ninety miles from Ottawa. The winters were so cold that buildings on campus were connected through a series of tunnels. But after two semesters with a roommate who constantly played Barry Manilow and of staring at farmland through her dorm room window, Ellen had enough. She transferred to Buffalo State, and we were together again.

While in school, my relationship with my father had begun to ease. I even saw flashes of remorse from him from time to time; while talking with my mother on the porch, he said quietly, "Jane, the divorce was all my fault. All of it."

Yet, most of the time I couldn't bring myself to ask him for help. Instead, I struggled to balance school, work, and helping my mother.

Despite annual inflation that approached double digits, Mom's alimony never rose. I gave her part of my paycheck every week, but she found it increasingly harder to pay bills on time. Mom's ten-year-old car had spots of rust from Buffalo's winters. Its aging frame and engine had one mechanical problem after another, including a leaky gas tank. I paid for a brand-new gas tank, but a month later, the transmission failed. *Doris Karloff*, as Mom dubbed it, met an ignoble end at a junkyard.

In winter, Buffalo's near-constant wind made it hard for her to breathe when she went out, so she mostly stayed in our dark, shabby house. The occasional humidity during the region's mild summers also caused breathing issues, so she would find no seasonal relief.

During an unusual heat wave in 1976, Mom began to gulp air compulsively. I quickly realized she needed an air conditioner. I wondered about talking over the problem with Dad, but pushed the thought away. Instead, I forked over the money to buy one. I didn't know purchasing power was leverage and a customer could insist on an immediate delivery.

So, when the sluggish sales clerk said the soonest delivery was in five days, I meekly agreed. The wait seemed endless as my mother panted like a dog. Finally, two men from the store delivered the behemoth, carrying it upstairs and installing it in Mom's bedroom window. When it roared to life, her breathing instantly improved.

Soon, she also had the hope of breathing easier over her finances. Her doctor suggested that she apply for a veteran's pension. He wrote a letter to the VA saying she was "permanently and totally disabled" because of her heart disease, and that she met the qualification for a non-service connected disability. The claims administrator who helped her apply also arranged for Mom's medals to be sent to her that she had earned during her service. When the six medals arrived, Mom solemnly pinned them on her bathrobe. We all laughed, and teased her, but were proud of her, nonetheless.

Yet, it would be months before the VA approved Mom's pension, and longer still before the first check arrived based on a stipend of about $180 a month. In the meantime, she fell further behind on bills. Unbeknownst to us, Mom hadn't paid the cottage taxes. And Sadie Hinkle, ever resentful of agreeing to sell the cottage to my mother, was waiting like a trap-door spider. More than anything, she wanted it back.

CHAPTER 45

DELINQUENT

EVERYONE IN NEWCOTT KNEW WHO WAS MORE THAN SIX MONTHS LATE PAYing taxes because town hall would post a list of delinquent properties. If an owner was more than a year late paying taxes, anyone could pay the tax bill and put in a bid to gain the property. The property wouldn't transfer to a new owner unless the bill went unpaid for several more years. When that happened, the property could be foreclosed upon and transferred to whomever had paid the taxes.

Sadie Hinkle would show up at town hall and pay mom's unpaid taxes while Mom struggled to scrape together the money.

Mom asked the tax office if she could pay part of the bill, and the clerk laughed.

"Lady, this isn't layaway. You have to pay the whole thing."

She avoided talking about it to us. She was ashamed, blaming herself for not doing a better job of juggling expenses. But her income, with alimony and her veteran's pension, never seemed to cover enough of the bills. Also, fewer of us kids lived at home to contribute to the household. Tim had moved to Australia for a teaching job; Seamus moved out to his own apartment; Ellen lived at home but didn't work, and Claudia had joined the Army as an officer. I took on more hours at work and increased the money I gave her, but it wasn't enough.

I noticed one morning that Mom was quieter than usual. She knew that the new list of tax delinquency was published that morning, and our cottage was on it. She hadn't paid the taxes in two years. She knew Sadie Hinkle would go to the town hall and plunk down a check for the tax bill. Then she would wait. Foreclosure loomed.

Later that afternoon, the phone rang. The caller was Bernice Bangs, part of the husband-and-wife team who had sold the cottage to Mom back in 1968, and now had a cottage three miles away, not far from Newcott. She invited Mom out to dinner.

"I don't know, Bernice," Mom said. "I don't really feel up to it."

But Bernice persisted.

"Bring Maura. Let's get dinner out, just the three of us."

Mom gave in, but still seemed uncharacteristically quiet as I helped her into the boat and pushed off from the dock. Across the harbor, I could see Bernice waiting. She had a navy blue, gleaming Cadillac, with leather seats. We glided to a town ten miles away.

The restaurant was deliciously cool in the summer heat. She encouraged us to have anything on the menu. I excused myself to go to the restroom. When I returned, Mom was animated. Her mood had changed.

Later, she told me what had taken place.

When I stepped away, Bernice opened her purse, took out a slip of paper, and handed it to Mom. The paper was the accumulated property tax bill for the cottage for the previous two years. Mom's name was at the top and the document was stamped PAID IN FULL.

Her friend's ever-present kindness brought tears to our eyes. The incident made me realize how close to the edge our finances were. I knew that money was a constant struggle, but I was clueless about the yearly taxes. I was so focused on the day-to-day expenses that I never realized how pressing property taxes could be, or how they loomed large to my mother.

It made me wonder what else I didn't know.

Plenty, as it turned out. That Christmas, I realized how bad things had gotten.

Dad had always given Mom more money than the court ordered him to pay, but there were some things that he just didn't consider a priority. Buying gifts, for example. That Christmas, he gave Mom a total of $50 to buy presents for us—$10 each, since Tim was in Australia. Mom used the money to pay other bills.

In the days before Christmas, we placed gifts on the mantel above the fireplace ahead of time but Mom hadn't put any on the mantel. On Christmas Eve, she closed the door of her bedroom, and I could hear her cutting wrapping paper. Finally, she emerged, arms piled high with presents. I tingled with anticipation as I saw them, wrapped in red, green, and gold. I wondered when she had managed to get to a mall.

We all began opening our gifts, and the room got quiet.

My present was a small, antique marble bust of a woman with her hair pulled up in a bun. It was lovely and I had admired it when Mom bought it years ago at an estate sale. It usually sat on her dresser.

Ellen got a small painting of Mom's.

Seamus got a dark, soft scarf that Mom usually wore around her neck in winter.

Each of us got a gift from Mom. But she hadn't bought any of them.

Finally, I began to see that increasing breathlessness wasn't all that discouraged her; it was her inability to afford what she longed to give to all of us—and simply couldn't.

Yet the lasting irony, so many decades later, is that all the material goods from childhood Christmases that once shone in department store windows or hung in proud display are dust. They are gone and forgotten. But I remember that Christmas, and I still have that beautiful marble bust on my office shelf that my mother gave me from the depths of her privation.

CHAPTER 46

ELLEN FINDS HER STRIDE

MOM'S HEALTH WAS SLIPPING, BUT ELLEN HAD BEGUN TO FIND HER RHYTHM. After all Ellen had gone through in childhood, she felt stunned to be alive. She and I began to run together for miles after our college classes and she gloried in her increasing strength. She also, finally, had an income of her own. Dad had helped her secure a job as a telephone operator thanks to one of the worst snowstorms ever to bury Buffalo—the blizzard of '77.

The blizzard remained legend in the city for decades. The freak weather system appeared without warning one January afternoon and pummeled the city for days. Buffalo residents take winter weather in stride, but this was an eye-opener—a life-threatening, four-day gale with constant wind and 70 mph gusts.

The winter had been unusually frigid. November had been the coldest in nearly a century. Lake Erie froze over completely by mid-December, a record, and it snowed virtually every day. Gigantic cliffs of powdery snow formed across the lake's vast expanse. As the blizzard slammed the area, a white wall of wind began pushing the towers of snow into defenseless Buffalo. Drivers trying to clear the streets couldn't see the plows at the front of their vehicles. Snow drifts buried houses. Cars were stranded and abandoned everywhere. People even froze to death seeking shelter.

Dad, as Red Cross disaster director for Western New York, had spent his career witnessing the devastation of nature's fury. Every year, he spent a week or two in a disaster area far from home. Tornadoes had chased him in Texas; hurricanes drenched him in Florida. His organizational abilities were honed by years of experience.

To combat the deadly storm, Dad assembled an army of volunteers, trucks, jeeps, and snowmobiles. The Red Cross's telephone operator couldn't make it in to work, though, and hundreds of phone calls went unanswered, so Dad enlisted Ellen to help. When her ride arrived, Ellen staggered through the howling wind to the vehicle. Before opening the car door, the skin around her nose and ears felt strange. Ellen put both her hands up and pulled away a perfect, frozen mask of her own face.

At the time, Seamus had introduced me to a friend who was moving to Florida and needed someone to share driving 1,400 miles. I was happy to escape winter for a week and blithely unaware of the impending crisis. However, in the following days, I watched national news about my hometown with growing horror. My brother Tim, sweltering during Australia's summer, was stunned to see a TV news report on the terrifying winter storm in faraway Buffalo.

As I sat beneath palm trees, Ellen taught herself the obscure workings of the General Electric PBX switchboard, with its lights, switches, and lengthy cords. Callers couldn't reach a department in the Red Cross unless Ellen pulled up a cord and jammed it into the right plug. During the blizzard, so many telephoned the organization for help that Ellen fielded six thousand phone calls, including one man who called in panic to say that his canary had flown out a window.

"Why the hell do you have a window open in this weather?" Ellen blurted out.

After the storm finally abated, Ellen proudly told me she only dropped three phone calls.

"Unfortunately," she chuckled, "it was the same guy three times."

After the storm, Ellen got a permanent job operating the switchboard. I doubted that she would show up at work on time, every day, but I couldn't have been more wrong. Ellen arrived early and stayed late. She never took a sick day. She also began to volunteer. She helped out on charity fundraisers and marathons. The following year, she managed school, a job, and volunteering, and best of all, realized her long-held ambition to row at the West Side Rowing Club.

I had always thought that the club admitting women as members was about as likely as women becoming priests in the Catholic Church. But then a catastrophe occurred, one which finally led to prying open doors to competitive rowing for women in Buffalo.

A rowing shell, with its thin, heavily varnished top surface, was improperly stored right-side up in the rafters of the clubhouse, too close to a light bulb. In the night, the shell began to smolder, sending sparks onto a gasoline can stored in a coach boat below. The resulting blaze reduced dozens of beautiful rowing shells to ashes. Seven remained unscathed only because several West Side crews were rowing at the annual Royal Canadian Henley Regatta twenty-five miles away. The club burned down.

Recovery, we knew, would take years.

But maybe, Ellen hoped, with the need to rebuild, the new building could make room for women.

Once the leaders of the club chose a new waterfront site, Ellen researched whether the land was public or private. In fact, the new site would require permits from government agencies.

Together, she and I wrote a letter to the city's corporate counsel, saying that the days when the West Side Rowing Club could shut the doors against women should be over—particularly if they built a new club on public land. Ellen was passionate on the subject. I cared more about the principle than the sport.

We never got a reply to our letter, perhaps because the change we wanted was already in the works.

The board of directors for the club held several meetings with club members, where they debated the pros and cons of admitting women. In the end, they concluded that building a new facility was the perfect moment to pivot. The vote to invite women to join was unanimous, and the club opened its doors to women in the spring of 1978. Ellen was among the very first to sign up and began training immediately.

CHAPTER 47

MOTHER'S DAY

WHILE ELLEN HAD ATTAINED HER LIFELONG DREAM OF ROWING, MOM'S breathlessness worsened. At the time, I wrote in my journal:

Every time Mom goes in the hospital, I think, "this is it."

She would always minimize the cause when she needed acute care. Once, she was incapacitated with a heart arrhythmia for several days. Another time she spent an entire week in the hospital.

But Mom encouraged me not to worry. She was a convincing actress, so it was easy to believe her. Hospitals had become a normal part of our lives through all those years with Ellen's illness, so Mom going to the hospital didn't faze me. She laughed away problems and downplayed her symptoms.

Meanwhile, I was consumed with my own desire to leave. Mom pushed me to think of my future as limitless. I desperately wanted to get away from home, from my responsibilities, and against all evidence to the contrary, decided my mother could manage without me for a while, so I signed up for an internship in Washington, D.C. My sister Kate was working on Capitol Hill, so I wouldn't be far from family.

Mom and I would write to each other every week. In her letters, she told me the winter cold made it almost impossible for her to leave the house, but conversations over the phone with friends cheered her up. And some of our young friends would stop by regularly to visit and keep her company while I was away.

As the cherry trees blossomed into pink clouds around Washington, and the last breath of winter blew in Buffalo, one of my internship supervisors told me I should go home for Mother's Day. But I argued it didn't make sense since I would be home two weeks later, when my internship ended.

"Do it anyway," she urged. "Your mama needs you."

I dismissed those comments. But both statements were true. My mother needed me. And I would be home for Mother's Day.

On May 5, Ellen called me. She sounded distracted and subdued.

"Hi, Maura, how are you?" she said.

I listened in disbelief.

"We have some mail for you here. The weather's been kinda cold."

There was a long pause, then Ellen spoke.

"Mom . . ." Another pause. "Mom . . ."

My panic rose.

"What's happening?" I interjected.

She tried again.

"Mom . . ."

"Mom had a heart attack." She nearly choked on her words. "It's been a tough winter. She's gone downhill. Maybe it would be better if she just let go."

And then she burst into tears.

Ellen was home at the time and called an ambulance. Mom slipped in and out of consciousness in the emergency room, but then heard the doctor tell my sister and my father she had just a few minutes to live. That woke her up. She crooked her finger at the doctor. Startled, he leaned over her and my mother hissed, loud enough for Ellen and Dad to hear:

"I am going to die . . . in a motorcycle accident . . . when I am ninety-two . . . with my FOURTH HUSBAND."

Then she lapsed into unconsciousness again.

I called an airline and reserved the last seat on a morning flight the next day. I spent the evening at Duddington's, a popular Capitol Hill watering hole, although I remembered none of it. I blacked out and woke up the following morning with a throbbing headache, my mouth desert-dry and all events after the phone call a complete blank.

Hungover, I caught the flight, and Dad met me at the airport. I was surprised to see him. I had expected one of my siblings to meet me in the terminal, but he told them he wanted to pick me up. He explained, as he drove me to Buffalo General Hospital, that Mom had pneumonia and heart failure.

Mom looked tiny, with IVs in her arms and a beeping machine tracking her heartbeat. Her face was gray and there were dark circles under her eyes. When I walked in, she struggled to sit up, weakly protesting:

"How's my baby? You came home early! You didn't have to. I'm not that sick—" A deep cough racked her body, and she couldn't finish her sentence.

"You sound just great," I said, putting up a cheerful front that I didn't feel. After a while, I told Mom to get some rest and assured her I would return in a few hours.

"She looks terrible," I said to Dad, waiting in the hall.

"You think so?" Dad said, grimly. "Well, she could pass a beauty contest compared to the way she looked yesterday."

We were both silent as he drove me home. The sight of my mother broke through my years-long denial regarding her health. *She is never going to get better*, I thought. As soon as I got home, I started to clean the house. The place was dark, dusty, and messy, a combination of Mom not having the energy to do housework and Ellen's perennial obliviousness to dirt or clutter.

How long did she have to live? I wondered, as I scrubbed the grimy floor of the front hallway. During the flush of Mom's inheritance, she had hired someone to cover the front hallway floor in off-white, marble-like tiles. They were beautiful when clean. But the tiles were nearly black when I began washing them. Gradually, their old color reappeared. I poured ammonia, soap, and water over the floor, mopping and squeezing out dark water into another bucket, brooding as I worked.

She had always looked forward to that bright future.

"Someday, at Thanksgiving, I will see the shining faces of my beautiful grandchildren around the table. You wait and see!"

Would Mom ever live to see any of us get married or have children? Would my children know her? Would they laugh on the sunporch of the cottage with their wisecracking grandmother? Would she teach them how to play rummy, insisting they are cheating if they won? Or cheer them on as they caught their first sunfish?

When I saw Mom the next day, I tried to hide how discouraged I was. But she sensed my mood immediately.

"What's wrong, honey?" she asked.

"All of this," I said, faltering, gesturing around the room at the machines, the tubes, the IVs. "I'm just so worried."

She nodded. Neither of us had the energy for pretense.

"Even if I am not in good health, at least I'm not in any pain," she said, quietly.

She was sitting up, but lay back down in her pillows, and coughed again, lifting a tissue to her mouth. As she pulled it away, I could see spots of blood.

Two days later, with Mom still in the hospital, I took a temporary job as a nurse's aide for a private patient in a nursing home. Midway through my shift, Ellen called again. Mom was failing. The head nurse guessed what was happening from my wide eyes and increasingly frantic responses to Ellen. She took the receiver from me and hung up.

"You go on," she said. "I'll take care of your patient."

I ran to the front door and sprinted eight blocks through the rain, mud spattering my white uniform. It was pouring. I arrived, soaked, and saw Ellen, Seamus, and Dad surrounding the pessimistic doctor, who we had nicknamed the Angel of Death.

"I've taken the liberty of calling for a priest. We've made her as comfortable as possible."

Dad started to cry. Wordlessly, Seamus put his arms around him in a bear hug.

And yet Mom hung on.

The hospital placed her on a ventilator, which hissed as it made her chest rise and fall, forcing oxygen into her still body. She lay in a coma.

I visited every day, sitting by her side, holding her limp, unresponsive hand for hours. My brothers and sisters, too, sat by her bed. We took informal shifts, knowing only one or two of us could be in her room at any one time.

One Saturday night, I arrived late in the evening. I asked a nurse how Mom was, and she shook her head.

"No change," she said. I nodded, and settled in beside Mom's bed and took her clammy hand in my own. Tubes were everywhere. She had tape on her cheeks around her mouth to hold steady the tube snaking down her throat. Her lips were dry. I dampened a washcloth and patted her mouth. The hours passed, and my head drooped further and further.

A nurse popped briefly into the room, smiled, and returned carrying a china cup filled with hot, strong black coffee perched on a delicate saucer. The smell, the cup, the simple act of kindness invigorated me. It was 2 a.m. I sipped from the cup and looked over to Mom. *This is how it all ends*, I thought. Few would see this little woman and guess how strong and determined she was.

I finished the coffee, set the cup and saucer aside and rested my head against the bedside rail.

Without warning, Mom's right hand clamped onto mine, with all the iron strength of decades of mixing clay for sculpture. This was not the frail grip of a dying woman. I jolted upright and looked at her.

She was smiling, her hazel eyes alive with joy.

She couldn't talk with the tube in her throat, but tapped a wrist as if she had a wristwatch. What was the time? Then she took my hand again and squeezed it.

I looked to see the clock, out of Mom's sight.

"It's 2:15 in the morning, Mom. You've been out for a long time."

She looked around, and pointed at the calendar on the wall.

"The date?" I asked. She nodded.

I turned to look at the calendar. Tears welled up in my eyes. I lifted her hand to my lips and kissed her fingers.

"Happy Mother's Day, Mom."

CHAPTER 48

SUMMER SKULLS

MOM CAME HOME AFTER THREE WEEKS IN THE ICU, BUT WAS STILL FRAIL. BIT BY bit, she began to recover, and my brothers and sisters began to go back to their lives. Claudia planned to move to the Washington area as well, with Mom's encouragement.

"Move to Washington. Find yourself a nice girl to date," she told Claudia.

That left Seamus, Ellen, and me.

Seamus was working full time and wanted to spend as much time as possible with his girlfriend Carol, whom he would later marry. Ellen planned to hone her skills at the West Side Rowing Club. That meant, in our family game of tag, I was it. There was nobody else to take care of Mom. I had only one goal: I wanted to bring her to the Island. If she could only get to her beloved Toad Hall, I knew she would get better. To do that, I needed money, but my unpaid internship had depleted my savings. I had to find work fast.

It wasn't easy to find a job in Buffalo in the late 1970s. With the decline of manufacturing, competition for any employment was fierce. A friend got me a job working at a candle manufacturer, well known for their holiday figurines. Employment at the factory peaked in late spring and early summer, while the plant manufactured candles for Halloween, Thanksgiving, and Christmas months in advance.

I worked on the Halloween assembly line. Every day, hundreds of glow-in-the-dark, grinning skulls marched inexorably down the line as far as the eye could see. Women from the East Side of Buffalo, who had worked at the plant for decades, wisecracked while effortlessly snatching the skulls off the line, wrapping them in cellophane in seconds and neatly boxing them for shipment.

"Louise, this one looks like your ex-husband," one shouted as she held up the gruesome Halloween specter.

"Naw, my husband never looked *that* good," Louise yelled back, and the ladies all hooted as the line supervisor told them to pipe down.

The ladies on the line were gazelles. I was a lumbering elephant. But they encouraged me.

"You'll get used to it, baby. College kids never keep up in the beginning," they said, winking at each other. By the end of the day, I was exhausted and felt like the village idiot. My clothes reeked of the fragrances that imbued the candles. As I waited for the bus, I smelled like a child who had raided her mother's entire perfume collection and emptied the bottles over her head.

The cottage will stay empty this summer, I thought, frustrated. I could not work full time and bring her to the cottage for just two days. She was too frail to go back and forth so often. Mom would have to spend the summer in the city, holed up in her bedroom. I needed time to be with her. I needed money. I could not have both.

When I entered the plant on my fourth day of work, I punched in ten minutes early, and dragged my feet to the assembly line and sat in a tall chair. My cackling co-workers gathered like hens in a barnyard. I noticed a man nearby, staggering as he got into a small forklift.

He ran the forklift in jerky movements, and the machine swung near where I was sitting. *Too close*, I thought.

"Hey buddy, watch it!"

Thirty seconds later the forklift slammed into the back of my chair and I hit the side of the assembly line before flipping over it. I wound up on my back staring at the factory ceiling.

There was silence, then chaos.

"He's drunk!"

"He hit the college kid!" ladies yelled.

"Help her up!" someone shouted. The line supervisor began to scream at the man who was still operating the weaving forklift. Workers surrounded me. A woman from the head office in high heels and a business suit appeared. She told me, coolly, that I could see the plant doctor right away.

The doctor, she told me, would help me return to work.

I was stunned. In that moment, I understood two things: my back and ribs ached slightly, but I was otherwise fine. And the solution to my problem of needing both time and money had arrived.

I asked for help to stand up. A dozen hands reached down. I turned to the lady from the office, who put a hand on my elbow to bring me to the medical clinic on site. I jerked my arm away.

"I'm seeing my own doctor. He'll decide when I can return to work."

I walked out the doors of the plant into the bright sunshine. The street was quiet. I could hear the hum begin within the factory. The skulls would roll down the line without my haphazard assistance for at least today, and maybe forever. When I walked in the house, Mom asked why I returned from work so early.

"I'm taking you to the Island," I replied. "But I need to make a few phone calls first."

I called a friend who had worked at the General Mills plant in South Buffalo and told him about my accident. He immediately understood what I was looking for.

"After a minor back injury, my doctor got me out of work for months," he laughed, then gave me the name of his physician. I made an appointment for the next day.

I worried that there was little to show in the way of injuries. I felt fine. My ribs were scraped, but I had gotten more banged up climbing trees. But the doctor gave my minimal bruising a cursory glance. He had seen it all before.

"Injuries of this nature take eight to ten weeks to heal," he said, and paused. Then he said, slowly and deliberately, "I hope you heard me."

The deal was obvious. I had to appear at the doctor's office to lie under a heat lamp for ten minutes three times a week. The doctor would bill the company. I would get a weekly worker's compensation check of about two-thirds of a week's pay.

The stack of forms I signed were our passport to the Island, where I knew Mom would recover.

CHAPTER 49

A LAST SUMMER

YET, GOING TO THE ISLAND WOULD NOT BE A LEISURELY ECHO OF PREVIOUS DAYS.

Mom was weak. I had to organize the cottage, and my life, to care for her. Fortunately, the years I spent working as a nurse's aide gave me the experience I needed.

The stairs leading from the dock to the cottage would be a nightmare, though.

"I'll manage somehow," she said, with all the bravado she could muster.

The location of the only bathroom was on the second floor. Mom wouldn't be able to manage the stairs multiple times a day.

Despite reluctance to ask my father for anything, I realized, finally, that I couldn't do it all. I called Dad and asked him to help me figure out what it would take to care for Mom. He seemed surprised and grateful, and told me to meet him at work. The Red Cross then had a supply closet that was a lending library of medical equipment. We agreed that it was time to raid it.

I met him at his office where he took me down a long corridor and unlocked the large room full of medical supplies. It was filled with wheelchairs and walkers, crutches, canes, a hospital bed, and portable toilets. We conferred. I didn't think Mom needed a walker, but I took one of the toilets. She would hate using it, but if I kept it in her first-floor bedroom, she could avoid having to walk up the stairs.

Another concern was humidity. Mom's breathing had gotten worse. Dad called Bernice Bangs, who immediately offered a used air conditioner, free, from her furniture store. He and I hauled it to the cottage. Now, all Mom had to do was get there.

When the time came, I helped ease her into a boat piled high with groceries, her clothes, and her books, and we motored across the harbor. She looked up at the stairs with a grim determination. She climbed up like a toddler, one careful step at a time, resting in between. Midway, she sat on the steps and looked out over the water. Then she began again. One step. Then another. I hovered, anxiously, ready to catch her if she fell. But finally, she reached the top and gazed upon her sanctuary—Toad Hall.

Mom turned to me in triumph, her eyes alight, even as her chest heaved from her exertions. I helped her into the sunporch, and she sank into her familiar wicker rocker.

"Put out the flag, Maura," she said, between gasps, "Let everyone know we are here. And, let's have a drink." I smiled and made both of us good, dark drinks—whiskey, water, and ginger ale—and brought them out to the sunporch. Mom was asleep, her head slumped on her chest. I let her nap for a while, then helped her, tottering, into the first-floor bedroom and tucked her in. She fell asleep immediately. I placed a bell within reach that she could use to call me.

I drank my whiskey. Then I drank hers. I listened to the murmur of the wind rustling the trees and the soft cooing of the mourning doves. We were here, at our healing refuge. My mother had never needed it more. And neither, perhaps, had I.

We fell into a rhythm that was at once familiar and yet also foreign. I had to go into the city three times a week to get heat treatments for my fake injuries. Fortunately, the doctor's office in Buffalo's Black Rock section was located across the street from a quiet neighborhood watering hole with 30 cent drafts. I made it a habit to stop by a half hour early for a beer—"a quick one," as my father would say. I never questioned my growing habit of imbibing even at noon.

I always drank after work to wind down when I worked as a nurse's aide, too, stopping by the Elmwood Restaurant, a block from home. George was almost always the bartender when I walked in after 11 p.m. He would pour me a shot of ouzo on the house before I even had a chance to sit down. The shot was the opening act of several hours of drinking, sometimes with friends from work. Once in a while, Mom would join us, walking the block from our house to the Elmwood Restaurant.

Those days when she could walk even a block seemed far away now, I thought, as I downed my Labatt draft and walked across the street to the doctor's office feeling a pleasant buzz. The effects had generally worn off by the time the treatment was over, which was just as well. I almost always had a long list of things to do before driving back to the cottage.

I would pick up Mom's prescriptions, make doctor's appointments for her, shop for groceries, do our laundry, pick up the mail, pay bills, stop by the bank, and, of course, buy a bottle of Fleischmann's Rye Whiskey whenever we got low on booze. (Both of us preferred the smoother taste of Canadian Club, but that was more expensive so, with mild regret, I stuck to Fleischmann's.)

Newport cigarettes, too, were essential. Mom had cut back significantly, but still smoked a few times a day. Mostly, she sucked on hard candies when she felt the urge to smoke in those years before nicotine gum. Her physician told her that her heart disease had advanced to the point that it would make no difference whether she smoked or not. I never questioned the fundamental insanity of this premise.

The effort of taking care of just one ailing person, even one who was as undemanding as my mother, was a constant revelation. How, I wondered, did she take care of the six of us when it took so much time, thought, and energy to take care of one human? How did she perform this non-stop work for years? Why didn't we ever notice the energy it took, to be housekeeper, cook, counselor, referee—to be a mother? Why did we take it all so for granted? Mom had sacrificed her own health and life for her children. Now she was as frail as some of the old ladies I had cared for as a nurse's aide. But they were in their eighties. Mom was just fifty-five.

Gradually, she got stronger. Still, she couldn't walk with me every evening to watch the sun set over Lake Ontario, our old ritual. That one-hundred-yard journey might as well have been a marathon. But she could sit on the sunporch.

Since our flag was out, neighbors stopped by.

Mrs. Crawley had decided to sell her cottage. This was to be her last summer after sixty-four years. At ninety, she was going to move to California to live with her daughter.

"I'm going to enroll in college," she said, her eyes bright. Neighbors planned a farewell party at the end of summer. Grace Cohen, at ninety-four, would try to attend.

"We'll be there," I promised.

As Mom got stronger, I thought she deserved a party, too, for her birthday—August 19th. Then everyone could stop by to see her. I began making plans.

Ellen wasn't at the cottage much. She was working out every day at the West Side Rowing Club with other women who had joined. To my surprise, the coaches and the "Old Boys" who ran the club welcomed the women with grace and humor. They threw themselves into teaching the new female members the fine points of rowing with energy, seriousness, and not a hint of reluctance. Even the once-recalcitrant Olympians who had competed in the 1936 Games pitched into coaching. Some of the male rowers, though, didn't like the change. Ellen endured their snide remarks without comment. She ran for miles and did sit-ups and push-ups before helping load the heavy workboat into the water. Mom smiled whenever we talked about her.

But more often, Mom dwelled on the long-ago past. She talked about her childhood, going to dance halls with her sisters and cousins, the years she spent during the war working at Curtiss-Wright Corporation on aircrafts, falling ill with encephalitis and, when she recovered, joining the Army. I listened. I sensed she wanted to explain her life to me—and to herself.

A few times that summer, I had to bring her to the city for her doctor's appointments. If the air was clear and the humidity low, we would cross the Peace Bridge to Ft. Erie, Ontario, and drive to Niagara Falls along the meandering and beautiful River Road, lined with lovely homes and grassy expanses next to the Niagara River. The American side was an eyesore lined with a six-lane highway, another tragedy of urban renewal that put cars ahead of people's right to enjoy the water. We avoided it. Instead, we drove through lovely old neighborhoods, admiring the nineteenth-century homes of Buffalo's Allentown section.

On one such outing, I drove us to Main Street and parked in front of Record Theatre, a storied local establishment in Buffalo. I turned to Mom and asked her to pick some music that she knew, but I had never heard. I would buy whatever record she picked.

"You're on," Mom said.

She tottered into the large store and entered the classical music section. The vinyl she selected wasn't Bach or Beethoven, but a composition by Aaron Copland, unknown to me, called "Appalachian Spring."

When we dropped the needle on the record that night, I thought it had the slowest beginning of any piece of music I had ever heard. After almost two and a half minutes, I opened my mouth to say something when Mom put her hand up, ever so slightly, her wordless message clear:

Wait. Just—wait.

Then I heard it: That stunning burst of violins uniting and cascading as one in a sudden, swirling dance of notes that, together, send one message: Joy.

I was transfixed. I listened to the composition over and over again. My enthusiasm made my mother smile.

"No matter what happens, you will always have 'Appalachian Spring,'" she told me.

The following week she was strong enough to water some annuals, making repeated trips between the kitchen faucet and the flower bed. Unexpectedly, she insisted on making dinner. I worried about her expending so much energy and kept trying to help until she barked in her best drill-sergeant tone, "Sit down!"

She waited on me, serving chicken, mushrooms, broccoli, and potatoes. After dinner, we walked to see Margaret McMann, who said her trademark "my stars!" putting her hand to her chest in surprise to see both of us.

Afterward, as I was shuffling cards for another game of rummy, Mom suddenly spoke.

"If I died, I hope you would go on with your life, that you wouldn't be too sad, for too long. I hope all you kids wouldn't just . . . scatter."

I tried to make a joke, but it was clear she was serious, even though it was obvious to me that she was getting better.

"You know, if you had died in May, I would have been a wreck. Everyone would have been a mess," I replied. "But now, I think we would be OK eventually. Sad, but OK."

"I'm glad," she said. "Now, deal."

The next afternoon, as I began to paint the back porch, Mom screamed.

I dropped the paintbrush and ran to her. She was gray, with cold sweat running down her face.

"I'm so nauseated," she said, over and over.

She had no pain at all, but she looked terrible, so I called 911. In a panic, I told the dispatcher who answered the phone that I thought she was having a heart attack.

"Please hurry."

In no time, volunteer firefighters and EMTs piled in a boat and roared across the harbor. The cottage filled with big men carrying a stretcher and medical equipment. Mom was sitting up, gasping for breath. A medic knelt beside her and nervously put his thumb on her wrist. Despite her condition, Mom laughed.

"You can't feel my heartbeat with your thumb, honey. That's *your* pulse you are feeling, not *mine!*"

They were the last words she said aloud. As she lost consciousness, the men loaded her on the stretcher and took her in an ambulance to a small community hospital seven miles away. I followed close behind. In no time, medical staff snaked a ventilator tube down her throat. The hissing began again. There would be no birthday party at the cottage.

I shoved dimes into the hospital pay phone, first calling the house in Buffalo, then Seamus's apartment, then Dad's apartment. I couldn't reach anyone but Ellen, who still had no drivers license and no way to get to the hospital. I told her to call our kind friend and Dad's former Red Cross colleague, Panky Curtiss. After Mom's May heart attack, she made me promise to call her if we ever needed help. Within minutes, Panky picked up Ellen and drove her fifty miles to the hospital. Ellen and I stayed at the hospital until evening, then went back to the cottage, turning in at ten. But soon, after just an hour of sleep, we were awakened by the shrill ringing of the telephone.

"Your mother's condition is critical. Come quickly," the voice said.

Unlike earlier in the day, when we arrived, Mom was awake, sitting up, clutching the side rails of the bed to stay upright. Her face lit up to see us and she settled back on the pillows, ventilator still in her mouth. Ellen brought a medal she had just won in a race and told Mom excitedly about all that she was learning at the rowing club. Mom, unable to speak, smiled and pretended to applaud.

Then Ellen leaned forward and asked, "Mom, do you love us?"

It was our teasing question from our childhood in the projects, which always brought the same answer. Mom smiled, nodded, and pointed up.

"Up to the ceiling," she was saying, her constant answer to us as children, when we could imagine nothing higher than the ceiling of our apartment.

We held her hands then, Ellen on one side, me on the other. And Mom's head began to droop. Time and again, she shook herself awake to look at us, smiling, gazing for long moments at me, then at Ellen. Ellen sensed what I did not, and leaned forward.

"Mom, hang on. Think about the shining faces of your grandchildren around the Thanksgiving table." Mom nodded, vigorously, her eyes joyful, but soon she became drowsy again.

Finally, she fell into a fitful sleep.

By that time, we had talked with her, off and on, for three hours.

She's not so bad, I thought. I asked a nurse why the hospital had summoned us. She lifted one eyebrow and gestured toward the bed.

"That was quite a performance," the nurse said. "I think she did everything she could to wait for you two."

"What do you mean?"

"Your mother has had no measurable blood pressure for five hours," the nurse replied.

By the next morning, she was comatose. Her eyes would flutter open, unseeing, then close again. She would turn her head one way, then the other. She moved her lips in unheard conversation. She seemed unaware of our presence. Her ever-enlarging heart still fluttered, but the shell of a body on the hospital bed no longer housed her radiant spirit.

She was dying.

I leaned over and kissed her eyes, her cheeks, and her forehead.

"Goodnight, darling," I whispered.

Mom twitched.

We were exhausted, and there wasn't much more we could do, so we drove back to the cottage and were finally able to reach everyone. I told Dad that I couldn't stay at the hospital anymore. I just couldn't stand it. Dad understood.

"I'll go," he said quietly. "She shouldn't die alone."

Ellen and I paced nervously, as we waited for the phone to ring, but it remained silent. By early evening, we were restless and decided to visit a neighbor a few doors away. Hal, a high school principal, welcomed us by wordlessly pouring mugs of cold draft beers from the taps in his living room. He made light conversation. I began to relax.

Soon, though, we heard howling just outside the door. Mom's giant Maine coon cat, Sara, adopted two years earlier from an animal shelter, had always been quiet and sweet. The gentle feline rarely even meowed for food. But here she was, caterwauling outside the cottage, pacing on the sidewalk, back and forth.

When I stepped out the door to try and quiet her, Sara immediately darted toward our cottage, and looked back at me expectantly. I stood, not moving. She scampered toward me, wailing, then turned around and ran twenty feet further, and turned to look back at me again. I went inside to where Hal and Ellen were sitting. Sara howled in response, ran back to Hal's cottage, and began scratching the door, clawing at the screen, on the verge of hysteria.

Ellen and I drained our mugs and walked outside, and Sara galloped ahead, leading us home. The phone rang as we entered. I picked up the receiver.

"Maura?" Dad said, in a voice very quiet and very old.

"Mom died," he whispered.

Ellen, watching me begin to weep, put her hands over her eyes.

"I'm glad you stayed with her, Dad. I just couldn't," I managed to say.

"I know, honey. I'll see you tomorrow."

"What? No. Don't drive back to the city tonight," I snapped back. "Stay here, with us."

Dad was silent for a moment.

"Are you sure?" he said, cautiously.

"You shouldn't be alone tonight, Dad. And, neither should we."

I had spent years hating him. But for all of Dad's infidelity during his marriage, he had been faithful to Mom at the end.

As I hung up the phone, I thought, Mom would never see the shining faces of her grandchildren. They would never hear her singing the aria from *Madama Butterfly* in the kitchen while she cooked.

Ellen and I walked out of the cottage, arms around one another. Infinite stars gleamed in the clear night. While our mother lay dying, a violent thunderstorm had swept through. Lightning and thunder crackled over Lake Ontario. The storm had cleansed the air of the thick humidity that made it so hard for her to breathe. We would never have to worry about that again. We stared up at the soaring river of the Milky Way. The Perseid meteor showers were just beginning. As if on cue, a diamond dropped from the sky and faded a moment later.

There she is, I thought.

I had never felt sadder, and yet, grief balanced with gratitude. My mother and I had long summer weeks together. That was a gift. I knew it would be the last summer I would ever spend so much time on the Island. But I was free now. And so was she.

I told myself that I was lucky to have had my mother for twenty years. It was unfair to lose her. But two decades was something, wasn't it?

What I feared the most, however, was not being able to say, "Last week, I said to Mom . . ." or "Just this past weekend, Mom and I . . ."

Soon it would be weeks, months, years, decades, I thought, desperately. Would I forget the sound of her voice?

"Oh, Ellen," I said, feeling as if I had swallowed broken glass. "How are we going to do this?"

"I don't know," she said, shaking her head. "I just don't know."

Chapter 50

Goodbyes

Mom's funeral was tiny. I wanted weeping crowds and a long line of people attesting to her warrior strength. I wanted public acknowledgment of her brilliance and her selflessness. I wanted news of her passing to be reported on television, with TV anchors nodding to one another and making small talk about the terrible loss. But reality was colder.

We paid for a death notice in the newspapers. There would be no separate news article; that was reserved only for men with careers and titles. The death of a divorced housewife with no career was nobody's idea of news.

Mom had insisted she wouldn't want her funeral to include a wake. I wanted us to follow her wishes, with no formal calling hours. I was too young to understand that funerals are for the living, not the dead. We should have had calling hours and a wake. And yet, it might have made the whole occasion even sadder. Few might have showed up. She died in the middle of August and everyone, it seemed, was on vacation. At the funeral Mass, the priest gave a generic, one-size-fits-all homily that made it plain that he had never met her and would not think of her ever again the moment he told us to "go in peace."

Peace, indeed. That was a joke.

Grief and guilt aged my father overnight. Dark circles appeared under his eyes. His hair seemed grayer. He didn't joke or tease, or even talk much. All he did was go to work or stay alone in his little apartment.

I began to worry about him. When I saw him, he was withdrawn and didn't say much. *Maybe he needs to be needed,* I thought. I called him.

"Dad, we should get the equipment back to the Red Cross, and return the air conditioner," I said, and he agreed.

We drove together to Newcott and crossed the harbor to the cottage. I cleaned equipment we had borrowed and packed a few of Mom's things, pausing to sob in her worn housedresses. Before we left, I stopped by Mrs. Crawley's going away party to wish her well.

Dad and I lugged the air conditioner onto the boat to return it to Mom's steadfast friend, kind Bernice Bangs. We loaded the machine onto the back of Dad's station wagon. He started the car and, before putting it in gear, pulled a quart bottle of Genesee Cream Ale out of a bag. He took a long pull and silently handed the bottle to me as he turned the car onto the country roads that would lead back to Buffalo. I gulped the beer and handed the quart bottle back to him. We passed the bottle back and forth as he drove. The bottle was empty long before we crossed the city line.

At night I experienced long hours of insomnia, spending my nights in a haze of walking through the house on Anderson Place, going to bars or sitting on the porch, joined by friends, or alone, a beer always at my side. My grief was a pulsating wound. I prayed for sleep that never came. Finally, one night, I wrapped myself in my mother's familiar bathrobe and crawled into her bed. I slept for fourteen hours in her bathrobe arms.

Warren Arthur, still aging, gaunt, and tall as ever, shuffled to our house from his funeral home across the street with Mom's ashes in a box under his arm. Under the other arm, folded in a triangle, was the American flag she had earned as a WWII veteran. He handed me the box. Then he handed Ellen the flag and she hugged it tightly to her chest, tears cascading down her cheeks. I realized then that if Mom had a more formal funeral, that my brothers, father, and other men would have escorted her coffin down the aisle of the church before her funeral Mass. Her coffin, unlike any other woman we knew, would have been draped proudly in the flag she had served in the Army. She should have had that much, I thought, with regret, as Ellen wept in the stars and stripes.

I looked at the box and shook it a little. I nearly dropped it, horrified to hear the rattling of the ashes and bits of bones. Ellen stopped crying and stared.

"Gee," she said after a moment's silence. "Mom sure doesn't look like herself."

We took the box to the little cemetery in Newcott where Mom and I had walked so often. She had a plot in a new section, under a sapling. I wished that her resting place was closer to the heart-shaped grave Mom and I had always visited during our walks. There, she could have kept little Mabel company. But Mabel lay in the oldest part of the cemetery, far from the newer plots. On the day we buried Mom, I visited Mabel first, brushed away leaves and said a silent prayer.

Then I walked to where Dad, a priest, Ellen, and Seamus stood. There was the headstone, with Mom's name, dates of birth and death, a Celtic cross and, proudly, "WWII" engraved upon it.

She would have liked that, I thought.

In the coming weeks, Dad sank further into the inky depths of sadness. When I called him, his voice was quiet and listless, and he ended the conversation after a few minutes. For a garrulous man who had spent his life socializing and telling stories, the transformation was shocking.

Ellen and I talked about Dad every day while running along Buffalo's waterfront. She had persuaded me to join her in a four-woman crew at the West Side Rowing Club. The workouts were a good distraction, but before and after, we talked about how much we missed Mom and how depressed Dad seemed to be. Yet, in spite of his depression, he quietly paid all the bills for the house so Ellen and I could continue to live at home.

The reasons I had hated him began to dissolve.

Finally, Ellen and I came to the same conclusion.

Dad should move home, we agreed.

We called him up and talked to him about moving back in the house he had not lived in for years. Dad was silent.

"Really?" he suddenly piped up with a mixture of disbelief and happiness.

"Yes," we said. "Really."

He became cautious.

"I want to move home," he said. "But I want to make sure you both want me. You think this over. I'll stay in my apartment for two months. If you still want me to move back, I'll do it," Dad said. "But if you don't, I'll understand."

Ellen and I both agreed. After two months, we had not changed our minds. Dad moved back into the house he and Mom had purchased together in 1964, the same house a restraining order forced him to leave.

Mom was gone. We were adults. Dad still drank, but I told myself that his alcohol use would matter less. I wasn't helpless. I wasn't a child.

Instead, I began to worry about Ellen's drinking.

CHAPTER 51

THE PRICE OF MOTHERHOOD

AFTER MOM'S DEATH, AND WHEN THE ROWING SEASON ENDED, ELLEN BECAME a binge drinker. Her alcohol use terrified me. She had begun to drink one afternoon when I decided the best way to slow her down was to take her to a movie, since colas and coffee were the only drinks then sold at movie theaters. (Ironically, in light of what happened next, the movie was *Animal House*.)

But Ellen had come prepared.

During the opening scene, Ellen opened the coat she was wearing to hide from the November chill, reached into the inside pocket, and pulled out a half-pint of vodka. She cracked open the top and began to drink the liquor, straight, like water. I lunged for the bottle and she tried to push me away. We began a noisy tug-of-war. I finally succeeded in ripping the bottle out of Ellen's clutches and put it securely under my seat, where she couldn't reach it.

Ellen was motionless for about two minutes. Then, without taking her eyes off the screen, she reached into one of the coat's side pockets and pulled out *another* half-pint of vodka, cracked it open, and began to drink. I reached for the second bottle and Ellen stiff-armed me as she slurped, the fiery liquid spilling out of the sides of her mouth. Finally, with other theatergoers threatening to call management, I gave up.

By the time the closing credits rolled at the end of the movie, Ellen was far drunker than she had been when she entered the theater. I got her home, somehow kept her from drinking any more, and held Ellen's head over the toilet as she began to purge her body. When she was spent, I helped her into bed and tucked her in. Exhausted, I went to bed, too. In the wee hours, I awoke to the too-familiar sounds of my childhood: Dad was stumbling around the kitchen, drunk, trying to make himself a meal. He slammed pans together and dropped a dish that shattered on the floor. He opened and shut the old refrigerator, with its safe-like door, repeatedly. Dad had gone on a bender. I stared at the ceiling, sleepless and disgusted.

The next day, both Dad and Ellen had the grandfather of all hangovers.

Pale and shaking, Ellen swore off booze, which sounded to me like an empty pledge.

Dad moaned, holding his head in misery.

They could both recover without me, I decided.

I packed an overnight bag and announced that I intended to drive to Cherry Creek, NY, to see our family friends, Irene and George.

Irene and George were friends of the family who, until retirement several years before, lived a few blocks away from us in an apartment they had rented for decades. After they moved away from the neighborhood, they encouraged visits, and so my mother and I made regular trips to see them every few months. We would drive through little towns, tiny dots on a map, and always stay overnight. I loved Irene, with her intelligent conversation and her distinctive voice, husky from years of smoking and mixing chemicals in the hair salon she owned. But I also knew how much she loved Mom, and that comforted me. I needed to get away.

"Feel better, Ellen," I called as I left.

"I hope so," she said in a tiny, shaky voice.

The drive brought memories of trips over the same green hills with Mom, before heart disease drained her energy and stole her life. Driving through the southern tier of New York State, near the border of Pennsylvania, was like going back in time. Serpentine byways curved around tumbledown barns and meadows, one vista lusher than the next. The few vehicles sharing the route included trucks piled high with hay, or a tractor hugging one side of the street while its driver waved me on. My body relaxed as I pulled into the driveway of their snug home. Their Labrador barked a warning, and I heard Irene's voice, saying, "George, who just pulled in?"

"Dunno, but I'll check."

As George emerged from the porch and saw me, he pulled his ever-present pipe out of his mouth.

"Oh, for Pete's sake. What are *you* doing here?" he asked, feigning anger.

"Go see Irene," he said, taking my bag. "She's been worried about you since your mother passed. Where's Ellen?"

"Long story," I called over my shoulder, and entered the house to Irene's waiting hug.

"You'll spend the night, of course," she ordered.

Irene had visited after Mom had come home from the hospital that previous June.

"Anyone could see that your mom was failing, honey."

I shook my head. "I knew she was sick, but I didn't think she would die."

Irene hesitated.

"Your mom knew that her time was limited."

"What do you mean?" I said.

"Remember when your mom visited us a little over two years ago? It was the only time I can remember that she came here alone, without one of you kids in tow."

I nodded. "It was after a doctor's appointment. She said she wanted to visit you alone."

"Yes," Irene said. "That was the day that Jane's doctor told her she had about two years to live. Your Mom drove here to talk about it. She asked if we would keep an eye on you and Ellen. Of course, I said we would. And, it seems the doctor was right. She lived one month short of two years after that day."

I was stunned. So Mom knew—every day, for two years until she died—that her heart was failing and time was slipping away. She knew she would soon die when she encouraged me to take an internship away from home. She knew her time was short when she insisted that Claudia should move to Washington, D.C. and "find a nice girl." She didn't say a word when Tim moved to New England for a job after teaching in Australia for two years.

"Why didn't she tell us?" I asked.

"Because she was a good mother," Irene retorted. "She didn't want you kids to hang around the house. She wanted you to live your lives. She would have hated holding you back. Any of you."

"But— but—" It was too much to take in. "Why did she get so sick? What started all this?"

"She always had a heart murmur. And, your lives weren't exactly calm for the last ten years, especially with Ellen being so sick and your dad's shenanigans," Irene retorted.

"If your mom didn't give her a kidney, Ellen would have died. You know that." She paused. "Most of all, your mother knew that. She would have done anything, absolutely anything, to save her life."

I had a sudden memory of how Mom spoke with satisfaction about badgering Ellen's doctors to let her donate her kidney. The doctors really didn't want to do it. They had fought it out behind closed doors. But Mom had prevailed. Why were the doctors so reluctant? Did they know something that we were never told?

"Did Mom—did the transplant start all this?" I asked Irene.

She hesitated.

"Jane's heart was never 100 percent," she said, finally. "And you know your mom. She would have done anything for any of you."

Irene, whose friendship I had prized for her bluntness and honesty, had evaded my question. But I didn't need her answer. I suspected that the kidney disease which had shattered Ellen's life and the scientific advances that had allowed my mother to donate her kidney had also contributed to my mother's early death at fifty-five.

I thought about all of this driving home the next day. Part of the route paralleled the shore of Lake Erie, the shallowest of the Great Lakes, where storms could spark enormous waves in far less time than it took to arouse deeper Lake Ontario. On this day, the water and the sky were both the color of steel. I turned off the road, parked the car and mulled over what I had learned.

Mom would have done whatever it took to save Ellen. I could imagine her desperation to give Ellen the gift of years, of realizing her dreams of rowing and living to adulthood.

Then came the doctor's warning that Mom had two years to live, and her solitary trip to Cherry Creek. Irene said that Mom was determined to tell no one of the doctor's pronouncement, least of all her children. I understood why. We could do nothing to fend off her fate. The knowledge of what was to come would have destroyed the last two years for everyone. None of us would have pursued our own ambitions. I would have hung around the house, staring at her.

Mom would have hated it.

Did I ever sense that her time was slipping away? Only once. Not long after that doctor's appointment, and her trip to Cherry Creek, Mom and I drove together to the Island. On that day, when we turned onto the country roads of Niagara County, she began to sing the sweet, sad African American spiritual, "Swing Low, Sweet Chariot." Mom always had a beautiful voice, but something in her heartfelt, melodious singing that day gave me pause. *She knows something*, I thought. It haunted me all that day.

Rain began to beat on the roof gently, then harder, obscuring my view of the water. I started the car, then turned on the windshield wipers.

"Oh, Mom," I said, "You were the strongest person I ever knew."

I turned the car out of the parking lot and drove home.

* * *

Despite the anguish over the loss fading as the years passed, my questions lingered. Finally, I tracked down Dr. Hawking, Ellen's physician, retired from medical practice in her native England. Her brother Stephen had become world famous for his genius, making it easy for me to find her. Within six hours of my sending an email, Dr. Hawking replied, with the subject line, "How lovely to hear from you." She was as kind and compassionate as I remembered. Through long conversations on Skype, the decades fell away. Finally, I asked her if the transplant contributed to Mom's heart disease and early death.

"Maura," she said leaning into the computer screen, "I *told* Jane well before the operation that it would damage her health. We all tried to dissuade her."

I brought up the same subject with Gay, one of our former neighbors at the projects, who was a young mother when we moved down the hall from her family's apartment. Mom loved Gay and talked to her regularly when Ellen was ill. In Gay's retirement home in Florida, I asked her the same question I asked Dr. Hawking.

"Absolutely," Gay replied immediately. "Doctors told her that the transplant would weaken her heart and drastically shorten her life."

"What did Mom say to that?"

"Your mother said, 'Oh, really? So just how healthy do you think my heart will be if my daughter dies?'"

CHAPTER 52

PETE

AFTER GRADUATING FROM COLLEGE, I WAS HIRED TO BE A CASEWORKER AT THE Salvation Army Men's Social Service Center in Kenmore, just outside Buffalo. Men could stay there if they remained sober and helped out at the Salvation Army stores and trucks, picking up donated clothes and furniture. The captain in charge hired me, irritating Peter Panzarella, who was the head of counseling at the Center. The captain had promised to leave employee decisions up to Pete, then hired me without consulting him.

"This here is Marsha," he blithely introduced me, getting my name wrong. "She'll start on Monday."

Pete stared at me. I stared back. I held out my hand to shake his. We disliked each other instantly.

Our mutual irritation would gradually diminish, though, as he and I worked to establish programs that helped men, then women, deal with drug addiction and alcoholism. Over the course of working together every day, we became ever closer. He was fascinated by addiction, but had no personal or family experiences with it.

After two years, we began to date. Pete was endlessly encouraging about my writing and helped me see that I could do more than just scribble in journals. With his gentle prodding, I began to apply to graduate schools for journalism. I moved to Washington, D.C. to attend American University and live with Claudia, who was then an Army officer. Pete drove eight hours from Buffalo to visit every two weeks during my year-long program, always arriving at around 11 p.m., tired but smiling, and always with a single rose in his hand for me. Soon, we became engaged.

We talked about our future together, and our families. While telling me about his mother's relatives, Pete told me that the Irish branch of my mother's family is named Dugan, but part of the family decided to put in an extra "g" in their names.

"Uh huh."

"So instead of Dugan, their last name is Duggan."

"OK . . . what about it?"

"Well, I think you know my cousin. She's a nun and taught at your high school."

My eyes widened.

"Sister Mary Kathleen Duggan?"

As Pete nodded, I felt a thrill. *If we have kids*, I thought, *they will be related to my most brilliant teacher, the one whose relentless optimism changed my life.*

"If I knew you were related to Sister Kathleen, I would have married you years ago," I said.

My father was delighted that Pete and I decided to get married. He loved the fact that Pete rarely drank.

"A son-in-law is the last person I want for a drinking buddy."

He asked what I wanted for a wedding gift.

"I only want one thing."

"I'll get you anything you want." He smiled.

"Don't get drunk on my wedding day."

My father's face fell, and he looked horrified.

After a moment, he looked at me earnestly and promised.

At the wedding party at the Island, he was the first to leave.

"If I stay, I'll get drunk," he said as he kissed me goodbye.

Chapter 53

"It's Dad."

A LITTLE OVER EIGHT YEARS LATER, IN 1987, THE PHONE RANG ON MY NEWS-room desk.

I was on deadline at *The Eagle-Tribune*, an afternoon daily newspaper in Lawrence, Massachusetts, just shy of forty miles from Boston. My title of Editorial Page Editor sounded more impressive than the reality of the job.

I expected this phone call to be another irate reader. Instead, Ellen was on the line.

"It's Dad," she said.

For Christmas dinner, he had a leg of lamb that he drenched in a wine marinade for two full days before roasting it. After gobbling the rich meal, helping himself to seconds and thirds, Dad began to have severe angina. His doctor ordered tests, and soon Dad underwent heart bypass surgery. A post-operative infection put him in the ICU and placed on a ventilator. His heart trouble was one result of his alcoholism. He cut back on his drinking after Mom died, but he still went on occasional benders.

By then, Ellen and I had both stopped drinking.

My alcohol use ended after I attended a journalism conference in Baltimore where I had promised myself that I wouldn't have more than two drinks but got drunk anyway. My loss of control scared the hell out of me and afterward, I never had another drink. Ellen made the same decision a year later, after being arrested for driving while intoxicated.

With my sister, I worried about more than our father's fate.

"Whatever happens with Dad, you know you can go to an AA meeting, right?" I said to Ellen.

"Yep. You too," she said.

After doctors took Dad off the ventilator, I finally decided to fly home.

As Ellen and I sat with him in his hospital room, the tube in his throat reduced his voice to a whisper. He asked us what had happened to him. His memory was spotty, so Ellen explained all of the complications from his surgery. Dad was silent for a few minutes, then suddenly, he gripped our hands and began to cry, tears rolling down his thin face. I thought that he might be upset about how many things had gone wrong.

He finally stopped, wiped his tears, and spoke, hoarsely.

"What would I have done without my kids? What would I have done without you kids here, at my side? Where would I be? *Who* would I be—without my children?"

Dad spent three months in the hospital. Spring came, then early summer. When he came home, he needed help getting shaved and taking showers. Pete and I decided we should spend a week in Buffalo so I could be with him.

When I walked into his bedroom, he looked gaunt. He had lost fifty pounds and was thinner than he had ever been. His gray hair had turned mostly white. He had become, to me, not just an old man. Dad wouldn't live to see autumn, I thought.

Surprisingly, the very taste of alcohol disgusted him. He abstained for the first time in fifty years. Even in the aftermath of his alcoholic scenes, my mother had always told us about how sweet my father had been when they dated, and in the early years of their marriage. Her memories had always struck me as euphoric recall, distortions of reality. I found it hard to believe that such a version of my father had ever existed.

But now, in sobriety, he had become a different person. Dad was kind, thoughtful, generous, and a good listener. I saw, finally, the man my mother had fallen in love with, and the father he might have been.

I loved being with this beautiful, reflective person. We talked and talked, and he told me about his bouts of insomnia.

"Why aren't you sleeping well? Is it the medication?"

Dad shook his head.

"I wasn't a good father," he whispered, his voice still hoarse from the ventilator. "I wasn't nice to your mother. I think of things that I shouldn't have done, but did anyway. Then I think about the things I should have done, and didn't."

"Oh, Dad. You have to sleep sometime. What helps?"

"I say the rosary," he said, holding up its beads made of Connemara marble and its silver Celtic cross. "I pray for forgiveness. I pray for your Mom. It's the only way I can get to sleep."

He hung his head, and we sat in silence for a moment, both at a loss.

"Your Mom. . . . I miss her so much," he continued. His eyes went past me and rested upon my wedding picture taken four years before. Pete and I stood in the center. Dad stood on one side, and Pete's parents stood on the other. Everyone is smiling in the sunshine, outside the church.

"I should have left a space," Dad whispered, gesturing at the picture.

"For what?" I said, confused.

"I should have left a space . . . for your mother."

* * *

One afternoon, Dad decided that he wanted Pete to take him for a drive. I was both insulted and pleased. Insulted that he didn't want *me* to drive, and instead, chose his son-in-law.

Pete helped Dad out of the house and eased him into his car. With me in the back seat, we took off on a bewildering tour. Dad gave directions that mystified me. We drove along the Lake Erie waterfront, through little towns outside Buffalo. But I couldn't figure out what Dad wanted so badly to see. It all seemed random.

Yet, Pete instinctively understood. Finally, he turned off the road and parked the car.

Pete turned to my father.

"You've helped a lot of people here, haven't you?" he said, gently.

"I've helped every single one of these people," Dad replied.

Then it was clear: The areas we drove through were located on flood plains.

He had, indeed, helped a lot of people through his Red Cross career aiding people after disasters. He wanted to remind himself that even if he had too often failed his family, his life had not been wasted.

At the end of the week, Pete and I drove back to Massachusetts.

Even though I had only told him that Pete and I intended to have a family someday, perhaps in a year or two, Dad told everyone that I was pregnant.

He told Ellen he couldn't wait to hold my baby.

"I have to get better," he said. "Maura and Pete will need help with the baby. I can cook and clean. I can take care of the baby during the day when they go back to work."

He outlined his plans with Ellen. If we didn't object, he could live with us for months. He wanted to be our live-in nanny.

"The baby can call me Granddad, like the whiskey." He winked.

Two weeks later, Ellen called at three o'clock in the morning to tell me that Dad had died in his sleep.

His funeral was everything we had wanted for our mother. His death was reported on the local evening TV news, with anchors nodding over Dad's legacy of helping people. It was the subject of an article in *The Buffalo News*. The wake was crowded. At his funeral Mass, his coffin was covered in the flag of the American Red Cross. A friend of mine sang the haunting melody of "A Parting Glass" while mourners wept:

Of all the money that e'er I spent
I've spent it in good company
And all the harm that ever I did
Alas, it was to none but me.

But since it falls unto my lot
That I should rise and you should not
I'll gently rise and softly call
Good night and joy be with you all.

Soon after the funeral, I began to experience food aversions. Tomatoes, which I always loved, suddenly repelled me. I felt nauseated every morning.

Maybe I just have some sort of flu, I thought. But I didn't have a fever. And I usually never felt sick. *Could it be?* I wondered. *Me, a mother?* It was hard to picture. *I'll feel better by the end of the week.* But Friday came, and the nausea continued.

After work, I stopped by a store to pick up cat food for a stray that had recently decided to adopt us. On the way to checkout, I saw home pregnancy tests for sale. I stopped and stared.

Nah, there's no way.

But, impulsively, I tossed a pregnancy test into my basket. Arriving home, my stomach churned at the sight of our many tomato plants, heavy with the red fruit. I put the box away in the back of a cabinet.

Ridiculous, I thought. *Waste of money.*

Despite my doubts, I took the test the next morning.

It turned pink. I laughed and laughed.

"Dad, you were right after all," I said aloud.

And I could almost hear his amused response.

"Granddad . . . like the whiskey."

CHAPTER 54

ELLEN AND ELLIE

AS I WATCHED MY GRANDDAUGHTER CLIMB ON THE OLD TOY, IT FELT AS THOUGH decades had passed in a heartbeat.

Pete and I had found the dusty, dimly-remembered rocking horse in the attic of our 250-year-old colonial home in Connecticut. The wooden horse was tucked in between a box of old papers from when he taught college and another box of clippings from the years I wrote editorials for *The New York Times*. The attic holds the bones of holidays past and the detritus of decades of marriage, two kids, and four moves.

Our daughter Anna had married and had become a mom of a feisty little girl. We thought our grandchild might like the wooden, painted rocking horse—which neither Anna nor her younger brother, Tim, ever played with much—so we cleaned it up.

As I watched, she sat on the horse and tottered furiously, back and forth. She loved it. Then, smiling, she scrambled onto the seat. She stood on it, and began to tilt on the wooden horse while, somehow, keeping her balance, shifting her weight, first on one foot, then the other, rocking in the riskiest way possible.

I was both horrified and amused. I edged closer to catch her in case she fell. I had a flash of memory: my daredevil sister Ellen, six years old, swinging back and forth on a high branch of a tree, and laughing.

"Ellie, be careful," I urged.

She is my sister's namesake, at Anna's kind insistence. Like Ellen, her first name is Elizabeth, but everyone calls her Ellie.

Once in a while, trying to keep up with her as she tears through the house, shouts orders at the dog, or runs away when I tell her it's time to eat or take a bath, I slip and call her Ellen.

My daughter Anna has only the dimmest memory of the aunt who died when she was three. Four years after our father passed away, Ellen's kidney, which had chugged along for twenty years against all odds and the doctors' predictions, finally began to fail. Ellen kept working full time at a hospital sleep clinic while she went back on dialysis. She stayed active as a volunteer coach at her beloved West Side Rowing Club, coaching scores of women rowers. Sometimes she relied upon unusual methods to pump up her crews before a race: One day she took out her fake eye and led the oarswomen in a dance around the plastic orb in the hopes of intimidating competing crews, who looked on, appalled. In her thirties, Ellen had become our family joke for her apparent inability to refuse any neighborhood Girl Scout selling cookies; she kept buying them even when she had seventy-five boxes piled in her basement chest freezer.

Ellen tried not to let her deteriorating condition slow her down, even administering dialysis to herself while driving across the country with Claudia, who, briefly, considered a job out West.

She tried to keep up her interests: scuba diving, coaching, and sailing the twenty-two-foot boat she docked at the cottage.

The drugs were more effective and treatment far more advanced than it was when we were kids. Yet, still, she was exhausted. She struggled to work full time.

Finally, she got a reprieve. A cadaver kidney became available from a young motorcyclist, killed in a November accident. The day of Ellen's second transplant, I was working as an editor at *The Day*, a newspaper in New London, Connecticut. I struggled to concentrate. I wrote my weekly column about my sister, my hopes for her, and the importance of organ donation, a topic I had visited time and again in my journalism career. While I wrote, I wept, not only in gratitude for Ellen's second chance, but for the broken hearts that young man whose kidney she was receiving had left behind. I marveled at the kindness of strangers.

Despite the successful transplant, complications from the procedure soon set in. They became too much for Ellen. Within two weeks, my sister's warrior heart finally stilled. We buried her on a bleak December afternoon, one day before her thirty-sixth birthday, next to our parents' graves in Newcott's small cemetery. Surrounding her fresh grave were the far more settled graves of those of many of our Island neighbors from summers we all once shared.

Christmas carols on the radio sang about joy and family gatherings. They mocked my grief.

I struggled to keep my sorrow from little Anna. Pete, always understanding, helped me go through the motions of the holiday. He sawed down an evergreen tree. We decorated it with my mother's ornaments. Anna chattered about the arrival of Santa Claus. She wondered which of the five fireplaces in our old colonial would he shimmy down? I was so far from the crumbling home of my childhood, and yet Ellen's death made me feel as though I were ten again—bewildered, defenseless, and lost.

Two weeks after Ellen's funeral, I was tucking Anna into bed when she grasped my hand, holding it tightly to her chest with both of her own.

"Mom," she said, her dark eyes looking into mine. "Don't be sad about Aunt Ellie. She was in our house last night."

My daughter's face lit up as she added: "And Aunt Ellie brought her mother here, too! Goodnight, Mommy, I love you."

She turned and fell asleep as I reeled, her words echoing in my head. For the first time in weeks, I smiled. A tiny seed of comfort grew in the pieces of my shattered heart. I thought of the joyous spirits of my sister and my mother visiting when I needed them the most.

Was it a dream? Who knows? Who cares?

"Oh, Mom. . . . Ellen." I took a breath. "Come back soon."

Now, thirty years later, my granddaughter Ellie and I stroll together through her quiet neighborhood. She picks up rocks and offers them to me as though they are diamonds. Back home, she runs and climbs. *She is not Ellen*, I remind myself, over and over. But, watching her, the decades fall away. Grief dissolves; I feel only gratitude. I have lived to see the shining face of my granddaughter. And through her, I catch glimpses of the sister I loved.

"Ellie, be careful," I say.

She laughs at my caution.

"No!"

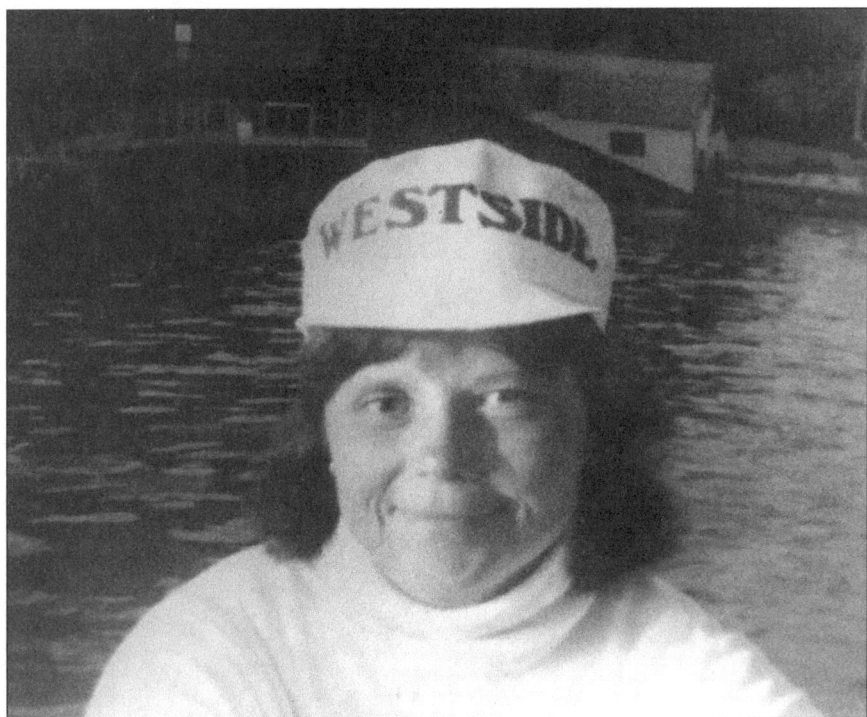

Ellen Casey
December 10th, 1955–December 5th, 1991

ACKNOWLEDGMENTS

I BEGAN WRITING THIS MEMOIR A FEW WEEKS BEFORE THE COVID PANDEMIC OF 2020. By the time lockdown started in the middle of March, I had written the first chapter.

For the next fourteen months I woke up at 5:30 a.m. and, with my beloved golden retriever, Molly, walked to my office on the second floor of our barn. There I read stacks of old diaries I had kept as a teenager. They were filled with dialogue, scenes and my mother's wisecracks, which still made me laugh. The diary entries jogged family memories, especially of my fearless and irrepressible sister Ellen. Some days, it felt as though my mother were pulling up a chair next to me and Ellen was helping me spell the big words.

While writing one's memories is always a subjective process, I tried to verify facts as well. I consulted old articles in *The Buffalo Evening News* and the *Courier Express*. I combed eBay for old postcards that made areas of Buffalo come alive again, such as beautiful Humboldt Parkway before it was destroyed to provide a faster route to the airport. Mark Goldman's wonderful books on Buffalo provided an historical perspective.

When I was done researching my beloved hometown, I examined the beginnings of the transplant field of which my sister played a small part. Old books of medical statistics and narratives from transplant pioneers helped. So did Dr. Glenn Geelhoed, who has conducted more than five hundred transplants starting in 1970, when he was in the Harvard Surgical Residency of the then-Peter Bent Brigham Hospital. He worked with Dr. Joseph E. Murray, the transplant pioneer and Nobel Prize winner who conducted the first kidney transplant in 1954. Glenn became a trusted resource and was always patient with my questions about the transplant field in the early days. I am also grateful to Angelo Zenez, who gave me an invaluable perspective on what it feels like to be on dialysis, and the mental and physical challenges of being a transplant patient. Kidney disease remains an agonizing battle for thousands of people. It takes courage to persevere and I salute the still-unappreciated and often-lonely struggle of patients and families.

The best reward of my research was tracking down and reconnecting with Dr. Mary Hawking, one of Ellen's doctors whose compassion was a bright spot during a difficult time. We were, in essence, time capsules for one another: She remembered me as a pesky eleven-year-old who walked her huge German Shepherd, Bran. I recalled her as a young physician who wasn't afraid to get to know her patients' families; she even took me to my first opera. Mary helped me with facts I couldn't pin down, and also confirmed medical details I could never have verified otherwise. The renewal of our friendship is an ongoing gift.

Readers will meet at the end of the book my sweet husband, Peter Panzarella, in the early days of our courtship and marriage. Pete encouraged me from the moment I told him I wanted to become a writer, when we were both working together in our twenties. He has been my rock through forty-plus years of marriage.

My daughter Anna and son Tim are central to my joy in life. They, along with my beloved brother Tim and sister Claudia, were so kind to read my book in early drafts.

My friend Roberta Baskin read excerpts of the book every week throughout the covid pandemic of 2020 and beyond, keeping me going through uncertainty. Connie Schultz, surely my bluntest friend and one of my dearest, helped me see that I was onto something in writing this book. Her support has meant the world.

One of the first authors whom I asked to read my book was Luanne Rice. Her early and kind support for my efforts brought tears to my eyes. J. Courtney Sullivan, Wally Lamb and Steve Kurczy were also more than generous with their time and encouragement.

Members of my tribe, the Mystic Writers, were generous in reading early drafts and giving me advice and guidance throughout the writing. Rosanne Hartman, an Anderson Place veteran, Ellen's best and most hilarious friend, read an early draft as did Gay Pye, our friend from the Buffalo projects, I am grateful for their friendship, and their love of my sister Ellen.

A total of twenty-eight people read the book, my so-called "beta readers" (whoever came up with that term?). They were to a person supportive and helpful. Thank you, all.

Thanks to my agent, Max Sinsheimer, of Sinsheimer Literary, who took a chance on me after thirty-four other agents either rejected my queries or ignored them. And, since every writer needs an editor, thank you to Skyhorse Publishing's Jesse McHugh, who cajoled, inspired, and pushed me to make this a better book.

Finally, although I have been at pains to assure the accuracy of what I have written, any memoir is subject to personal interpretation and the imperfect prism of memory. Those are mine alone and I do not mean for the scenes and events in these pages to speak for anyone else but me.

TO MY READERS

IF YOU HAVE GOTTEN THIS FAR, YOU HAVE INVESTED CONSIDERABLE TIME IN reading this portion of my family's history. I am grateful that you have walked with me in this journey. I am available on zoom for book clubs and would be happy to hear your thoughts on the book. You can email me by going to my website, www.caseyink.com, and hitting one of the "contact" buttons at the end of each page.

It would mean a great deal to me if you would leave a review of my book on Amazon, Goodreads, or whatever site suits you. Reviews, even short ones no longer than a sentence or two, help books gain traction in this too-crowded market, and give authors valuable feedback. Love it or not, I'm always interested in what readers think of my work. Thank you again for spending time with my story.

BIBLIOGRAPHY

Altman, Lawrence K. Antigens may prove key to organ transplantation, NYT, October 11, 1980, page 7.

Batterman, Nancy, Esq. Truro Law Review, Volume 10, number 3, 1994, *Under age: A minor's right to consent to health care.*

Barker, Clyde F. And Markmann, James F., *Historical overview of transplantation,* Cold spring harbor perspectives in medicine, April 2013.

Braun, W.E., Dausset, J., Jeannet, M. Fifteen years of HL-A: What is the importance of HL-A compatibility for clinical outcome of renal transplantation? Vox Sn 1978; 34:171–188 (248,Terasaki).

DiFonzo, J. Herbie and Stern, Ruth C.. Addicted to Fault: Why Divorce Reform Has Lagged in New York State, 27 Pace Law Review, 559 (2007)

Goldman, Mark, *High Hopes: The Rise and Decline of Buffalo, N.Y.* Albany, NY State University of New York Press, 1983.

Goldman, Mark, *City of My Heart, Buffalo 1967–2020,* Buffalo, Friends of the Buffalo Story, 2021.

Iniotaki-Theodoraki, A. The role of HLA class I and class II antibodies in renal transplantation. Nephrology Dialysis Transplantation, 2991.

Langhoff, E. and B.K. Jakobsen, et al, The impact of low donor-specific MLR versus HLA-DR compatibility on kidney graft survival, Transplantation, 1985 Jan; 18–21.

Lucas, Zoltan J. Renal Transplantation—Cadaveric Donor and Current Results with Renal Transplantation, Related Donors, The Western Journal of Medicine, March 1971.

Martin, Donald C., Renal Transplantation Results, Western Journal of Medicine, April, 1970.

Mezrich, Joshua D., M.D. *When Death Becomes Life: Notes from a Transplant Surgeon*, NY, NY Harper Collins, 2019.

Pilpel, Harriet, *Minors' rights to medical care, 1971.*

Sadler, Blair L. and Alfred H. Jr., Organ Transplantation and the Uniform Anatomical Gift Act: A Fifty Year Perspective, Hastings Center Report, March-April 2018.

Schlich, Thomas (2011), The art of medicine: The origins of organ transplantation, The Lancet, Vol. 378, 1372–1373.

Terasaki, Paul I. (1985), *Clinical Kidney Transplants 1985*, UCLA Tissue Typing Laboratory, LA, Calif.

Terasaki, Paul I., Editor, *History of Transplantation: Thirty-Five Recollections*, 1991, The Regents of the University of California.

Tilney, Nicholas L., M.D. *Transplant: From Myth to Reality*, New Haven, Yale University Press, 2003.

Stats on kidney donation in the United States since 1988 (500,000-plus) from the Organ Procurement and Transplantation Network.